Fundamentals of Nursing

Fundamentals of Nursing

Edited by
Yvonne Cowell

Larsen & Keller
www.larsen-keller.com

Fundamentals of Nursing
Edited by Yvonne Cowell
ISBN: 978-1-63549-709-0 (Hardback)

© 2018 Larsen & Keller

☰ Larsen & Keller

Published by Larsen and Keller Education,
5 Penn Plaza,
19th Floor,
New York, NY 10001, USA

Cataloging-in-Publication Data

Fundamentals of nursing / edited by Yvonne Cowell.
    p. cm.
Includes bibliographical references and index.
ISBN 978-1-63549-709-0
1. Nursing. 2. Care of the sick. 3. Medical care. I. Cowell, Yvonne.
RT41 .F86 2018
610.73--dc23

For more information regarding Larsen and Keller Education and its products, please visit the publisher's website www.larsen-keller.com

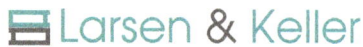

Table of Contents

Preface

Nursing as a profession deals with the care of families, communities and individuals. It includes the practice of helping each person so that they feel healthy, both mentally and physically. Nurses are an integral part of the healthcare system, they work closely with doctors, patients, physicians, therapists, etc. Their work includes helping in diagnosing problems, providing therapy and prescribing medication. This book is a compilation of chapters that discuss the most vital concepts in the field of nursing. It presents the complex subject in the most comprehensible and easy to understand language. This textbook is an essential guide for both academicians and those who wish to pursue this discipline further.

To facilitate a deeper understanding of the contents of this book a short introduction of every chapter is written below:

Chapter 1- Nursing is a part of health care sector which focuses on the wellbeing of individuals or families in order for them to maintain optimal health. Nurses provide care holistically to a patient and develop a plan of treatment. This chapter will provide an integrated understanding of nursing.

Chapter 2- Nursing theory is the development of techniques and facilities to improve the care of patients. Adaptation model of nursing, Levine's conservation model for nursing, Neuman systems model, self-care deficit nursing theory and Roper–Logan–Tierney model of nursing are some of the theories discussed in the following chapter. This chapter elucidates the crucial theories and principles of nursing.

Chapter 3- The different types of nursing are surgical nursing, flight nurse, obstetrical nursing, nurse anesthetist, peranesthesia nursing and certified nurse midwife. Surgical nurse provides care to the patient during the surgery and after it as well. Obstetrical nurses are nurses who work with women who are pregnant or are trying to conceive. The major types of nursing specialties are dealt with great details in the chapter.

Chapter 4- The management of the employment of nurses is known as nursing management. Some of the processes included in nursing management are organizing, directing, staffing and controlling. Nurse licensure, nurse uniform, nurse-led clinic and nurse–client relationship are the topics explained in the chapter. The aspects elucidated in this chapter are of vital importance, and provide a better understanding of nursing management.

Chapter 5- Health care is concerned with the diagnosis, treatment and prevention of illnesses, injuries and disorders. It encompasses professional health care services as well as care provided at the home. It varies from country to country and mainly depends on the economical condition of the nation. This chapter is an overview of the subject matter incorporating all the major aspects of health care.

I would like to share the credit of this book with my editorial team who worked tirelessly on this book. I owe the completion of this book to the never-ending support of my family, who supported me throughout the project.

Editor

Introduction to Nursing

Nursing is a part of health care sector which focuses on the wellbeing of individuals or families in order for them to maintain optimal health. Nurses provide care holistically to a patient and develop a plan of treatment. This chapter will provide an integrated understanding of nursing.

Nursing

Nursing is a profession within the health care sector focused on the care of individuals, families, and communities so they may attain, maintain, or recover optimal health and quality of life. Nurses may be differentiated from other health care providers by their approach to patient care, training, and scope of practice. Nurses practice in many specialisms with differing levels of prescriber authority. Many nurses provide care within the ordering scope of physicians, and this traditional role has shaped the public image of nurses as care providers. However, nurses are permitted by most jurisdictions to practice independently in a variety of settings depending on training level. In the postwar period, nurse education has undergone a process of diversification towards advanced and specialized credentials, and many of the traditional regulations and provider roles are changing.

Nurses develop a plan of care, working collaboratively with physicians, therapists, the patient, the patient's family and other team members, that focuses on treating illness to improve quality of life. In the U.S. (and increasingly the United Kingdom), advanced practice nurses, such as clinical nurse specialists and nurse practitioners, diagnose health problems and prescribe medications and other therapies, depending on individual state regulations. Nurses may help coordinate the patient care performed by other members of an interdisciplinary health care team such as therapists, medical practitioners and dietitians. Nurses provide care both interdependently, for example, with physicians, and independently as nursing professionals.

Nursing historians face the challenge of determining whether care provided to the sick or injured in antiquity was nursing care. In the fifth century BC, for example, the Hippocratic Collection in places describes skilled care and observation of patients by male "attendants", who may have been early nurses. Around 600 BC in India, it is recorded in Sushruta Samhita, Book 3, Chapter V about the role of nurse as "the different parts or members of the body as mentioned before including the skin, cannot be correctly described by one who is not well versed in anatomy. Hence, any one desirous of acquiring a thorough knowledge of anatomy should prepare a dead body and carefully, observe, by dissecting it, and examine its different parts."

Before the foundation of modern nursing, members of religious orders such as nuns and monks often provided nursing-like care. Examples exist in Christian, Islamic and Buddhist traditions amongst others. Phoebe, mentioned in Romans 16 has been described in many sources as "the first visiting nurse". These traditions were influential in the development of the ethos of modern nursing. The religious roots of modern nursing remain in evidence today in many countries. One example in the United Kingdom is the use of the honorific "sister" to refer to a senior nurse.

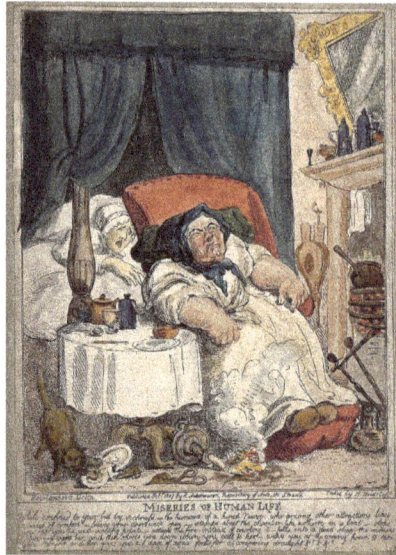

A convalescing woman trying in vain to rouse her slumbering hired nurse: the cat scavenges her food and the candle sets light to the carpet. Coloured etching by Nikolaus Heideloff (de), 1807, after Thomas Rowlandson

During the Reformation of the 16th century, Protestant reformers shut down the monasteries and convents, allowing a few hundred municipal hospices to remain in operation in northern Europe. Those nuns who had been serving as nurses were given pensions or told to get married and stay home. Nursing care went to the inexperienced as traditional caretakers, rooted in the Roman Catholic Church, were removed from their positions. The nursing profession suffered a major setback for approximately 200 years.

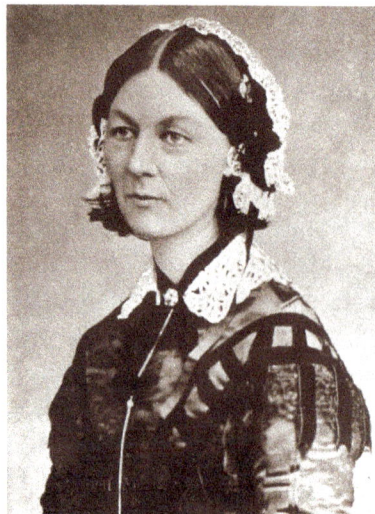

Florence Nightingale was an influential figure in the development of modern nursing. No uniform had been created when Florence Nightingale was employed during the Crimean War. Both nursing role and education were first defined by Florence Nightingale

Florence Nightingale laid the foundations of professional nursing during the Crimean War. Her *Notes on Nursing* became popular. The Nightingale model of professional education, having set up the first school of nursing that is connected to a continuously operating hospital and medical school, spread widely in Europe and North America after 1870.

Other important nurses in the development of the profession include:

- Agnes Hunt from Shropshire was the first orthopedic nurse and was pivotal in the emergence of the orthopedic hospital The Robert Jones & Agnes Hunt Hospital in Oswestry, Shropshire.

- Agnes Jones, who established a nurse training regime at the Brownlow Hill infirmary, Liverpool, in 1865.

- Linda Richards, who established quality nursing schools in the United States and Japan, and was officially the first professionally trained nurse in the US, graduating in 1873 from the *New England Hospital for Women and Children* in Boston

- Clarissa Harlowe "Clara" Barton, a pioneer American teacher, patent clerk, nurse, and humanitarian, and the founder of the American Red Cross.

- Saint Marianne Cope, a Sister of St Francis who opened and operated some of the first general hospitals in the United States, instituting cleanliness standards which influenced the development of America's modern hospital system.

Catholic orders such as Little Sisters of the Poor, Sisters of Mercy, Sisters of St. Mary, St. Francis Health Services, Inc. and Sisters of Charity built hospitals and provided nursing services during this period. In turn, the modern deaconess movement began in Germany in 1836. Within a half century, there were over 5,000 deaconesses in Europe.

Formal use of nurses in the modern military began in the latter half of the nineteenth century. Nurses saw active duty in the First Boer War, the Egyptian Campaign (1882) and the Sudan Campaign (1883).

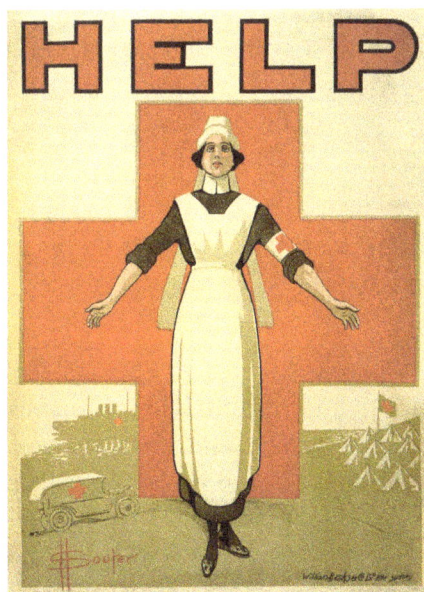

A recruiting poster for Australian nurses from World War I.

Hospital-based training came to the fore in the early 1900s, with an emphasis on practical experience. The Nightingale-style school began to disappear. Hospitals and physicians saw women in nursing as a source of free or inexpensive labor. Exploitation of nurses was not uncommon by employers, physicians and educational providers.

Many nurses saw active duty in World War I, but the profession was transformed during the second World War. British nurses of the Army Nursing Service were part of every overseas campaign. More nurses volunteered for service in the US Army and Navy than any other occupation. The Nazis had their own Brown Nurses, 40,000 strong. Two dozen German Red Cross nurses were awarded the Iron Cross for heroism under fire.

The modern era saw the development of undergraduate and post-graduate nursing degrees. Advancement of nursing research and a desire for association and organization led to the formation of a wide variety of professional organizations and academic journals. Growing recognition of nursing as a distinct academic discipline was accompanied by an awareness of the need to define the theoretical basis for practice.

In the 19th and early 20th century, nursing was considered a women's profession, just as doctoring was a men's profession. With increasing expectations of workplace equality during the late 20th century, nursing became an officially gender-neutral profession, though in practice the percentage of male nurses remains well below that of female physicians in the early 21st century.

Definition

Although nursing practice varies both through its various specialties and countries, these nursing organizations offer the following definitions:

Nursing encompasses autonomous and collaborative care of individuals of all ages, families, groups and communities, sick or well and in all settings. Nursing includes the promotion of health, prevention of illness, and the care of ill, disabled and dying people. Advocacy, promotion of a safe environment, research, participation in shaping health policy and in patient and health systems management, and education are also key nursing roles.

—International Council of Nurses

The use of clinical judgment in the provision of care to enable people to improve, maintain, or recover health, to cope with health problems, and to achieve the best possible quality of life, whatever their disease or disability, until death.

—Royal College of Nursing (2003)

Nursing is the protection, promotion, and optimization of health and abilities; prevention of illness and injury; alleviation of suffering through the diagnosis and treatment of human responses; and advocacy in health care for individuals, families, communities, and populations.

—American Nurses Association

The unique function of the nurse is to assist the individual, sick or well, in the performance of those activities contributing to health or its recovery (or to peaceful death) that he would perform unaided if he had the necessary strength, will or knowledge.

— Virginia Avenel Henderson

As a Profession

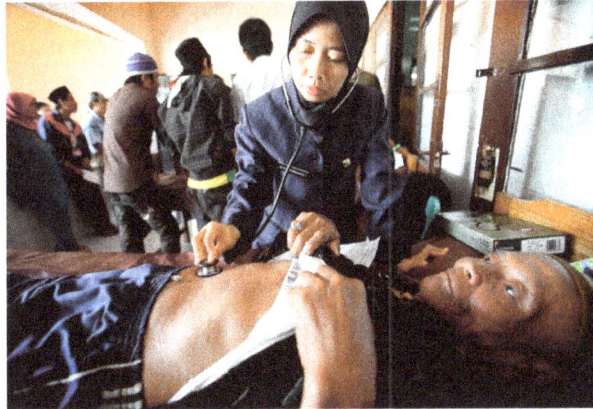
A nurse in Indonesia examining a patient

The authority for the practice of nursing is based upon a social contract that delineates professional rights and responsibilities as well as mechanisms for public accountability. In almost all countries, nursing practice is defined and governed by law, and entrance to the profession is regulated at the national or state level.

The aim of the nursing community worldwide is for its professionals to ensure quality care for all, while maintaining their credentials, code of ethics, standards, and competencies, and continuing their education. There are a number of educational paths to becoming a professional nurse, which vary greatly worldwide; all involve extensive study of nursing theory and practice as well as training in clinical skills.

Nurses care for individuals of all ages and cultural backgrounds who are healthy and ill in a holistic manner based on the individual's physical, emotional, psychological, intellectual, social, and spiritual needs. The profession combines physical science, social science, nursing theory, and technology in caring for those individuals.

To work in the nursing profession, all nurses hold one or more credentials depending on their scope of practice and education. A licensed practical nurse (LPN) (also referred to as a licensed vocational nurse, registered practical nurse, enrolled nurse, and state enrolled nurse) works independently or with a registered nurse (RN). The most significant differentiation between an LPN and RN is found in the requirements for entry to practice, which determines entitlement for their scope of practice. For example, Canada requires a bachelor's degree for the RN and a two-year diploma for the LPN. A registered nurse provides scientific, psychological, and technological knowledge in the care of patients and families in many health care settings. Registered nurses may earn additional credentials or degrees.

In the United States, multiple educational paths will qualify a candidate to sit for the licensure examination as a registered nurse. The Associate Degree in Nursing (ADN) is awarded to the nurse who has completed a two-year undergraduate academic degree awarded by community colleges, junior colleges, technical colleges, and bachelor's degree-granting colleges and universities upon completion of a course of study usually lasting two years. It is also referred to as Associate in Nursing (AN), Associate of Applied Science in Nursing (AAS), or Associate of Science in Nursing (ASN). The Bachelor of Science in Nursing (BScN) is awarded to the nurse who has earned an American four-year academic degree in the science and principles of nursing, granted by a tertiary education university or similarly accredited school. After completing either the LPN or either RN education programs in the United States, graduates are eligible to sit for a licensing examination to become a nurse, the passing of which is required for the nursing license. The National Licensure Examination (NCLEX) test is a multiple choice exam nurses take to become licensed. It costs two-hundred dollars to take the NCLEX. It examines a nurses ability to properly care for a client. Study books and practice tests are available for purchase.

Nurses may follow their personal and professional interests by working with any group of people, in any setting, at any time. Some nurses follow the traditional role of working in a hospital setting. Other options include: Pediatrics, Neonatal, Maternity, OBGYN, Geriatrics, Ambulatory, or Nurse Anesthetists. There are many other options nurses can explore depending on the type of degree and education acquired. RNs may also pursue different roles as advanced practice registered nurses.

Nurses are not truly doctor's assistants. This is possible in certain situations, but nurses more often are independently caring for their patients or assisting other nurses. Registered Nurses treat patients, record their medical history, provide emotional support, and provide follow-up care. Nurses also help doctors perform diagnostic tests. Nurses are almost always working on their own or with other nurses. Nurses will assist doctors in the emergency room or in trauma care when help is needed.

Gender Issues

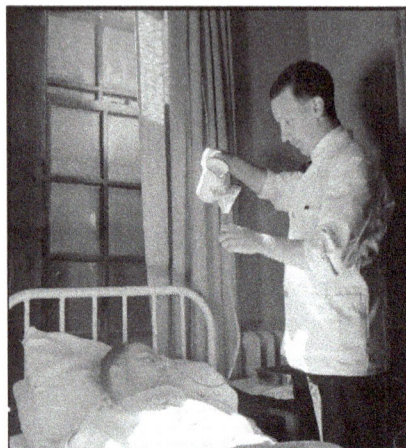

A male nurse at Runwell Hospital, Wickford, Essex, in 1943

Despite equal opportunity legislation, nursing has continued to be a female-dominated profession. For instance, the male-to-female ratio of nurses is approximately 1:19 in Canada and the United States. This ratio is represented around the world. Notable exceptions include Francophone Africa, which includes the countries of Benin, Burkina Faso, Cameroon, Chad, Congo, Côte d'Ivoire, the Democratic Republic of Congo, Djibouti, Guinea, Gabon, Mali, Mauritania, Niger, Rwanda, Senegal, and Togo, which all have more male than female nurses. In Europe, in countries such as Spain, Portugal, Czech Republic and Italy, over 20% of nurses are male. The number of male-registered nurses in the United States between 1980 and 2000s doubled.

There are many myths about nursing, including the profession and the people that work as a nurse. One of the most common myths is that all nurses are females. The nursing industry is dominated by females, but there are male nurses in the profession as well. A study in 2011 shows that 91% of all nurses in the United States were female, and 9% were male. Although females are more common, male nurses receive more pay. In the same survey, male nurses average $60,700 per year and female nurses average $51,100 per year. Male nurses have the highest percentage as nurse anesthetists, rating at 41%.

Theory and Process

Nursing practice is the actual provision of nursing care. In providing care, nurses implement the nursing care plan using the nursing process. This is based around a specific nursing theory which is selected based on the care setting and population served. In providing nursing care, the nurse uses both nursing theory and best practice derived from nursing research.

In general terms, the nursing process is the method used to assess and diagnose needs, plan outcomes and interventions, implement interventions, and evaluate the outcomes of the care provided. Like other disciplines, the profession has developed different theories derived from sometimes diverse philosophical beliefs and paradigms or worldviews to help nurses direct their activities to accomplish specific goals.

Scope of Activities

Activities of Daily Living Assistance

Assisting in activities of daily living (ADL) are skills required in nursing as well as other professions such as nursing assistants. This includes assisting in patient mobility, such as moving an activity intolerant patient within bed. For hygiene, this often involves bed baths and assisting with urinary and bowel elimination.

Medication

Nurses do not have the authority to prescribe medications, with few exceptions. All medications administered by nurses must be from a medication order from a licensed practitioner. Nurses are legally responsible for the drugs they administer and there may be legal implications when there is an error in a drug order and the nurse could be expected to have noted and reported error. In the United States, nurses have the right to refuse any medication administration that they deem to be harmful to the patient. In the United Kingdom there are some nurses who have taken additional specialist training that allows them to prescribe certain medications.

Patient Education

The patient's family is often involved in the education. Effective patient education leads to fewer complications and hospital visits.

Specialities

Nursing is the most diverse of all healthcare professions. Nurses practice in a wide range of settings but generally nursing is divided depending on the needs of the person being nursed.

The major populations are:

- communities/public
- family/individual across the lifespan
- adult-gerontology
- pediatrics
- neonatal
- women's health/gender-related
- psych/mental health

There are also specialist areas such as cardiac nursing, orthopedic nursing, palliative care, perioperative nursing, obstetrical nursing, oncology nursing, nursing informatics, telenursing.

Practice Settings

Nurses practice in a wide range of settings, from hospitals to visiting people in their homes and caring for them in schools to research in pharmaceutical companies. Nurses work in occupational health settings (also called industrial health settings), free-standing clinics and physician offices, nurse-led clinics, long-term care facilities and camps. They also work on cruise ships and in military service. Nurses act as advisers and consultants to the health care and insurance industries. Many nurses also work in the health advocacy and patient advocacy fields at companies such as Health Advocate, Inc. helping in a variety of clinical and administrative issues. Some are attorneys and others work with attorneys as legal nurse consultants, reviewing patient records to assure that adequate care was provided and testifying in court. Nurses can work on a temporary basis, which involves doing shifts without a contract in a variety of settings, sometimes known as *per diem nursing*, *agency nursing* or *travel nursing*. Nurses work as researchers in laboratories, universities, and research institutions. Nurses have also been delving into the world of informatics, acting as consultants to the creation of computerized charting programs and other software.

Occupational Hazards

Internationally, there is a serious shortage of nurses. One reason for this shortage is due to the work environment in which nurses practice. In a recent review of the empirical human factors and ergonomic literature specific to nursing performance, nurses were found to work in generally poor environmental conditions. Some countries and states have passed legislation regarding acceptable nurse-to-patient ratios.

The fast-paced and unpredictable nature of health care places nurses at risk for injuries and illnesses, including high occupational stress. Nursing is a particularly stressful profession, and nurses consistently identify stress as a major work-related concern and have among the highest levels of occupational stress when compared to other professions. This stress is caused by the environment, psychosocial stressors, and the demands of nursing, including new technology that must be mastered, the emotional labor involved in nursing, physical labor, shift work, and high workload. This stress puts nurses at risk for short-term and long-term health problems, including sleep disorders, depression, mortality, psychiatric disorders, stress-related illnesses, and illness in general. Nurses are at risk of developing compassion fatigue and moral distress, which can worsen mental health. They also have very high rates of occupational burnout (40%) and emotional exhaustion (43.2%). Burnout and exhaustion increase the risk for illness, medical error, and suboptimal care provision.

In the United States, the Occupational Health Safety Network (OHSN) is an electronic surveillance system developed by the National Institute for Occupational Safety and Health (NIOSH) to address health and safety risks among health care personnel, including nurses. It focuses on three high risk and preventable events:

- Musculoskeletal injuries from patient handling activities;
- Slips, trips, and falls
- Workplace violence

Hospitals and other healthcare facilities can upload the occupational injury data they already collect for analysis and benchmarking with other de-identified facilities, in order to identify and implement timely and targeted interventions.

Nurses are also at risk for violence and abuse in the workplace. Violence is typically perpetrated by non-staff (e.g. patients or family), whereas abuse is typically perpetrated by other hospital personnel. 57% of American nurses reported in 2011 that they had been threatened at work; 17% were physically assaulted.

Prevention

There are a number of interventions that can mitigate the occupational hazards of nursing. They can be individual-focused or organization-focused. Individual-focused interventions include stress management programs, which can be customized to individuals. Stress management programs can reduce anxiety, sleep disorders, and other symptoms of stress. Organizational interventions focus on reducing stressful aspects of the work environment by defining stressful characteristics and developing solutions to them. Using organizational and individual interventions together is most effective at reducing stress on nurses.

Worldwide

Australia

Catholic religious institutes were influential in the development of Australian nursing, founding many of Australia's hospitals - the Irish Sisters of Charity were first to arrive in 1838 and established St Vincent's Hospital, Sydney in 1857 as a free hospital for the poor. They and other orders like the Sisters of Mercy, and in aged care the Sisters of the Little Company of Mary and Little Sisters of the Poor founded hospitals, hospices, research institutes and aged care facilities around Australia.

A census in the 1800s found several hundred nurses working in Western Australia during the colonial period of history, this included Aboriginal female servants who cared for the infirm.

The state nursing licensing bodies amalgamated in Australia in 2011 under the federal body AHPRA (Australian Health Practitioner Registration Authority). Several divisions of nursing license is available and recognized around the country.

- Enrolled nurses may initiate some oral medication orders with a specific competency now included in national curricula but variable in application by agency.

- Registered nurses hold a university degree (enrolled nurses can progress to registered nurse status and do get credit for previous study)

- Nurse practitioners have started emerging from postgraduate programs and work in private practice.

- Mental health nurses must complete further training as advanced mental health practitioners in order to administer client referrals under the *Mental Health Act*.

Australia enjoys the luxury of a national curriculum for vocational nurses, trained at TAFE colleges or private RTO. Enrolled and registered nurses are identified by the department of immigration as an occupational area of need, although registered nurses are always in shorter supply, and this increases in proportion with specialization.

In 1986 there were a number of rolling industrial actions around the country, culminating when five thousand Victorian nurses went on strike for eighteen days. The hospitals were able to function by hiring casual staff from each other's striking members, but the increased cost forced a decision in the nurses' favor

European Union

In the European Union, the profession of nurse is regulated. A profession is said to be regulated when access and exercise is subject to the possession of a specific professional qualification. The regulated professions database contains a list of regulated professions for nurse in the EU member states, EEA countries and Switzerland. This list is covered by the Directive 2005/36/EC .

Iran

Nursing educational program in Iran is similar to the nursing educational program in other countries from some aspects. Holding secondary school diploma and passing the entrance exam is necessary for the admission in this course. Entrance exam to governmental universities and Azad University is held on separate basis. Duration of associate degree course of operating room and anesthesia is 2 years, bachelor's degree in nursing is 4 years and master's degree in nursing is 2-2.5 years and PhD degree in nursing is 4–5 years.

In the beginning, nursing educational program was the part of medical educational program. On the basis of this structure, the nurse follows the instruction of physician without any question. Nowadays, nursing educational program in Iran has been progressed and after the year 1992 considering the community base care, the nursing educational program also has changed. At present nursing education is held in 43 governmental nursing colleges and 63 nursing colleges of Azad University. Governmental universities' students do not have to pay tuition fee, but in Azad University, which is a private university, the students must pay necessary expenses. The PhD degree program is held only in governmental universities under the supervision of Ministry of Health and Ministry of Sciences.

In bachelor's degree program, nursing students start the clinical work from 2nd term and pass till the completion of 6th term simultaneously with theoretical subjects. 7th and 8th terms are allocated for training program. At present nursing educational program in throughout Iran is the same and is compiled under the supervision of Supreme Council of Ministry of Health, Treatment and Medical Education. Nursing students take the theoretical subjects, training and internship courses in various sections of educational hospitals and hospitals that affiliated to universities. Students' learning, in clinical sections is performed under the direct supervision and guidance of nursing instructors, but in the final year, activities of students mainly performs under the supervision of nursing personnel and alternate supervision of nursing instructors.

Students, during the years of study have opportunity to create relation with patients in the various sections especially intensive care units and to achieve experiences. Students' progress in clinical environments is from simple issues toward harder issues. At present practical nursing degree and associate degree Nursing Program has been canceled and Iranian nurses must hold bachelor's degree to work in Iran from accredited universities confirmed by the Ministry of Health.

Nursing Groups

- Nurse

Nurse is a person who is holding four years university degree and executes works relating to nursing profession including taking care of patients, perform health and medical services, educational, research and managerial affairs. At present annually 6000 persons are graduated in the bachelor's degree program in nursing.

- Practical Nurse

A person who is holding secondary school diploma in nursing and have completed 2 years program in nursing and cooperate in activities of nurses in medical sections under the supervision of nurses.

- Nursing Assistant

A person who is holding secondary school diploma and passing short term program for the execution of initial cares of patients under the supervision of nurses.

- Operating Room Technician

These persons after obtaining secondary school diploma and passing university's entrance exam and completing 2 years program are in charge of performing professional duties in operation room for preparing patients for surgery and necessary cooperation with surgeons at the time of surgery. These persons by passing the exam are eligible to continue uncontinuous bachelor's degree course in nursing.

- Anesthesia Technician

These persons after obtaining secondary school diploma and passing university's entrance exam and completing 2 years program in Anesthesia, are in charge of performing profession duties in the operating room in the field of anesthesia including preparing the patients for anesthesia and necessary cooperation with anesthesiologists at the time of operation. These persons by passing exam are eligible to continue uncontinuous bachelor's degree course in nursing.

- Emergency medical technician

These persons after obtaining secondary school diploma and passing entrance exam of university and obtaining technician diploma are in change of performing affairs including rendering first aid services to the patients and emergency victims resulting from accidents with motor vehicles, explosion, debris, falling from height, fractures, burns, poisonings, cuts, drowning, industrial accidents (cutting of limbs), patients with heart diseases and baby delivering.

- Master in Nursing

Nurses after obtaining bachelor's degree and passing the entrance exam are eligible to continue their study in geriatric nursing, pediatric nursing, medical surgical nursing, community health nursing, psychiatric nursing and nursing education. These persons after graduation mainly become in charge of nurses' education or management of medical sections. Duration of this program is 2.5 years. At present annually 150 persons are graduated in master's degree program in nursing.

- PhD in Nursing

Nurses by holding master's degree after passing entrance exam, are eligible to continue their study in PhD in the field of Nursing. Duration of this program is 4 years and the graduates mainly will work in educational and research sections. At present annually 20 persons are graduated in this program.

Nursing Jobs

According to the censes at present approximately 120,000 nurses are working in Iran in various sections. Most of them are working in hospitals and health centers belong to Ministry of Health, Treatment & Medical Education. Also, nurses are working in the hospitals affiliated to social security organization, armed forces, private sector and charity sector.

Within the last years of independence, nurses' activities are established in offices of consultancy and rendering nursing services at home. Nurses by establishment these centers can render consultant and care services to the client.

At present to work as a nurse only holding accredited academic degree is sufficient, but there are programs for nurses to take RN examination after graduation.

Also, upon the approval and execution of continuous educational act, the Iranian nurses should obtain score of 15 every year in various educational courses held by the Ministry of Health of Universities, Scientific Associations and Nursing organization.

Iranian Nursing Organization (INO)

Having an independent organization that defends the rights of nurses and to follow up nurses' problems was the long time wishes of Iranian nurses. Before Islamic revolution in 1979, efforts in this respect finally led to the establishment of the Iranian Nurses Association and activities were taken in this respect. After the victory of Islamic revolution, this association also canceled its activities and after that, number of associations mainly with political and professional formation was established, but the main problem of nurses was still present. Gradually in the year 1994 with the efforts of numbers of persons mostly nursing students and faculty member, the preliminary step was taken for the establishment of nursing organization. This preliminary nucleus started its work in the name of Nursing Coordination council with the instruction of students.

This council had correspondences with the president, speaker of parliament, ministry of health, treatment and medical education in connection with problems of nursing society. Also this organization had correspondence with nursing colleges for unity throughout the country.

After this date till March 2001, a number of state seminars were held in various cities and finally on March 5.2001, generalities of formation of Nursing Organization was entered in the agenda of the Islamic Consultative Assembly, and finally approved in an open session on Aug.12.2001. Finally with the procurement of comments of Guardian's Organization in Jan.2002, Establishment Act of Nursing Organization was approved by the parliament.

The first election of board of directors throughout the country was performed on Sept.20.2002 and members of 85 boards of directors of districts were elected throughout the country with the direct vote of nurses. The board of directors of the first Supreme of Organization, was elected on Dec.8.2002.

United Kingdom

To practice lawfully as a registered nurse in the United Kingdom, the practitioner must hold a current and valid registration with the Nursing and Midwifery Council. The title "Registered Nurse" can only be granted to those holding such registration. This protected title is laid down in the Nurses, Midwives and Health Visitors Act, 1997. From April 2016, nurses in the United Kingdom are expected to revalidate every three years.

First and Second Level

First-level nurses make up the bulk of the registered nurses in the UK. They were previously known by titles such as RGN (registered general nurse), RSCN (registered sick children's nurse), RMN (registered mental nurse) and RNMS (registered nurse (for the) mentally subnormal). The titles used now are similar, including RNA (registered nurse adult), RNC (registered nurse child), RNMH (registered nurse mental health) and RNLD (registered nurse learning disabilities).

Second-level nurse training is no longer provided, however they are still legally able to practice in the United Kingdom as a registered nurse. Many have now either retired or undertaken conversion courses to become first-level nurses. They are entitled to refer to themselves as registered nurses as their registration is on the Nursing & Midwifery Council register of nurses, although most refer to themselves as ENs or SENs.

Advanced Practice

- Nurse practitioners – Most of these nurses obtain a minimum of a master's degree, and a desired post grad certificate. They often perform roles similar to those of physicians and physician assistants. They can prescribe medications as independent or supplementary pre-scribers, although are still legally regulated, unlike physician's assistants. Most NPs have referral and admission rights to hospital specialties. They commonly work in primary care (e.g. GP surgeries), A&E departments, or pediatrics although they are increasingly being seen in other areas of practice. In the UK, the title "nurse practitioner" is legally protected.

- Specialist community public health nurses – traditionally district nurses and health visi-tors, this group of research and publication activities.

- Lecturer-practitioners (also called practice education facilitators) – these nurses work both in the NHS, and in universities. They typically work for 2–3 days per week in each set-ting. In university, they train pre-registration student nurses, and often teach on specialist courses for post-registration nurses

- Lecturers – these nurses are not employed by the NHS. Instead they work full-time in uni-versities, both teaching and performing research.

Managers

Many nurses who have worked in clinical settings for a long time choose to leave clinical nursing and join the ranks of the NHS management. This used to be seen as a natural career progression for those who had reached ward management positions, however with the advent of specialist nursing roles, this has become a less attractive option.

Nonetheless, many nurses fill positions in the senior management structure of NHS organizations, some even as board members. Others choose to stay a little closer to their clinical roots by becom-ing clinical nurse managers or *modern matrons.*

Nurse Education

Pre-registration

To become a registered nurse, one must complete a program recognised by the Nursing and Mid-wifery Council (NMC) . Currently, this involves completing a degree, available from a range of universities offering these courses, in the chosen branch specialty, leading to both an academic award and professional registration as a 1st level registered nurse. Such a course is a 50/50 split of learning in university (i.e. through lectures, assignments and examinations) and in practice (i.e. supervised patient care within a hospital or community setting).

These courses are three (occasionally four) years' long. The first year is known as the common foundation program (CFP), and teaches the basic knowledge and skills required of all nurses. Skills included in the CFP may include communication, taking observations, administering medication and providing personal care to patients. The remainder of the program consists of training specific to the student's chosen branch of nursing. These are:

- Adult nursing.

- Child nursing.

- Mental health nursing.

- Learning disabilities nursing.

As of 2013, the Nursing and Midwifery Council will require all new nurses qualifying in the UK to hold a degree qualification. However, those nurses who hold a diploma, or even a certificate in nursing are still able to legally practice in the UK, although they are able to undertake university modules to obtain enough credits to top up to a degree.

Midwifery training is similar in length and structure, but is sufficiently different that it is not considered a branch of nursing. There are shortened (18 month) programs to allow nurses already qualified in the adult branch to hold dual registration as a nurse and a midwife. Shortened courses lasting 2 years also exist for graduates of other disciplines to train as nurses. This is achieved by more intense study and a shortening of the common foundation program.

As of 2016 student nurses in the UK can apply a bursary from the government to support them during their nurse training, and may also be eligible for a student loan, although there has been speculation that this will not be available in the future.

Before Project 2000, nurse education was the responsibility of hospitals and was not based in universities; hence many nurses who qualified prior to these reforms do not hold an academic award.

Post-registration

After the point of initial registration, there is an expectation that all qualified nurses will continue to update their skills and knowledge. The Nursing and Midwifery Council insists on a minimum of 35 hours of education every three years, as part of its post registration education and practice (PREP) requirements.

There are also opportunities for many nurses to gain additional clinical skills after qualification. Cannulation, venipuncture, intravenous drug therapy and male catheterization are the most common, although there are many others (such as advanced life support), which some nurses undertake.

Many nurses who qualified with a diploma choose to upgrade their qualification to a degree by studying part-time. Many nurses prefer this option to gaining a degree initially, as there is often an opportunity to study in a specialist field as a part of this upgrading. Financially, in England, it was also much more lucrative, as diploma students get the full bursary during their initial training, and employers often pay for the degree course as well as the nurse's salary.

To become specialist nurses (such as nurse consultants, nurse practitioners etc.) or nurse educators, some nurses undertake further training above bachelor's degree level. Master's degrees exist in various healthcare related topics, and some nurses choose to study for PhDs or other higher academic awards. District nurses and health visitors are also considered specialist nurses, and to become such they must undertake specialist training. This is a one-year full-time degree.

All newly qualifying district nurses and health visitors are trained to prescribe from the Nurse Prescribers' Formulary, a list of medications and dressings typically useful to those carrying out these roles. Many of these (and other) nurses will also undertake training in independent and supplementary prescribing, which allows them (as of 1 May 2006) to prescribe almost any drug in the British National Formulary. This has been the cause of a great deal of debate in both medical and nursing circles.

Canada

Canadian nursing dates all the way back to 1639 in Quebec with the Augustine nuns. These nuns were trying to open up a mission that cared for the spiritual and physical needs of patients. The establishment of this mission created the first nursing apprenticeship training in North America. In the nineteenth century there were some Catholic orders of nursing that were trying to spread their message across Canada. Most nurses were female and only had an occasional consultation with a physician. Towards the end of the nineteenth century hospital care and medical services had been improved and expanded. Much of this was due to Nightingale's influence. In 1874 the first formal nursing training program was started at the General and Marine Hospital in St. Catharines in Ontario.

Education

All Canadian nurses and prospective nurses are heavily encouraged by the Canadian Nurses Association to continue their education to receive a baccalaureate degree. They believe that this is the best degree to work towards because it results in better patient outcomes. In addition to helping patients, nurses that have a baccalaureate degree will be less likely to make small errors because they have a higher level of education. A baccalaureate degree also gives a nurse a more critical opinion, which gives him or her more of an edge in the field. This ultimately saves the hospital money because they deal with less problematic incidents. All Canadian provinces and territories except for the Yukon and Quebec require that all nurses must have a baccalaureate degree. The basic length of time that it takes to obtain a baccalaureate degree is four years. However, Canada does have a condensed program that is two years long.

Nursing specialty certification is available through the Canadian Nurses Association in nineteen practice areas. Some of those specialties are cardiovascular nursing, community health nursing, critical care nursing, emergency nursing, gerontological nursing, medical-surgical nursing, neuroscience nursing, oncology nursing, orthopedic nursing, psychiatric/mental health nursing, and rehabilitation nursing. Certification requires practice experience and passing a test that is based on competencies for that specialty.

Public Opinion

Canadian nurses hold a lot of responsibility in the medical field and are considered vital. According to the Canadian Nurses Association, "They expect RNs to develop and implement multi-faceted plans for managing chronic disease, treating complex health conditions and assisting them in the transition from the hospital to the community. Canadians also look to RNs for health education and for strategies to improve their health. RNs assess the appropriateness of new research and technology for patients and adjust care plans accordingly".

Japan

Nursing was not an established part of Japan's healthcare system until 1899 with the Midwives Ordinance. From there the Registered Nurse Ordinance came into play in 1915. This established a legal substantiation to registered nurses all over Japan. A new law geared towards nurses was created during World War II. This law was titled the *Public Health Nurse, Midwife and Nurse Law* and it was established in 1948. It established educational requirements, standards and licensure. There has been a continued effort to improve nursing in Japan. In 1992 the Nursing Human Resource Law was passed. This law created the development of new university programs for nurses. Those programs were designed to raise the education level of the nurses so that they could be better suited for taking care of the public.

Types of Nurses

Japan only recognizes four types of nursing and they are Public Health Nursing, Midwifery, Registered Nursing and Assistant Nursing.

Public Health

This type of nursing is designed to help the public and is also driven by the public's needs. The goals of public health nurses are to monitor the spread of disease, keep vigilant watch for environmental hazards, educate the community on how to care for and treat themselves, and train for community disasters.

Midwifery

Nurses that are involved with midwifery are independent of any organization. A midwife takes care of a pregnant woman during labour and postpartum. They assist with things like breastfeeding and caring for the child.

Nursing Assistant

Individuals who are assistant nurses follow orders from a registered nurse. They report back to the licensed nurse about a patient's condition. Assistant nurses are always supervised by a licensed registered nurse.

Education

In 1952 Japan established the first nursing university in the country. An Associate Degree was the only level of certification for years. Soon people began to want nursing degrees at a higher level of education. Soon the Bachelor's degree in Nursing (BSN) was established. Currently Japan offers doctorate level degrees of nursing in a good number of its universities.

There are three ways that an individual could become a registered nurse in Japan. After obtaining a high school degree the person could go to a nursing university for four years and earn a bachelor's degree, go to a junior nursing college for three years or go to a nursing school for three years. Regardless of where the individual attends school they must take the national exam. Those who attended a nursing university have a bit of an advantage over those who went to a nursing school. They can take the national exam to be a registered nurse, public health nurse or midwife. In the cases of become a midwife or a public health nurse, the student must take a one-year course in their desired field after attending a nursing university and passing the national exam to become a registered nurse. The nursing universities are the best route for someone who wants to become a nurse in Japan. They offer a wider range of general education classes and they also allow for a more rigid teaching style of nursing. These nursing universities train their students to be able to make critical and educated decisions when they are out in the field. Physicians are the ones who are teaching the potential nurses because there are not enough available nurses to teach students. This increases the dominance that physicians have over nurses.

Students that attend a nursing college or just a nursing school receive the same degree that one would who graduated from a nursing university, but they do not have the same educational background. The classes offered at nursing colleges and nursing schools are focused on more practical aspects of nursing. These institutions do not offer many general education classes, so students who attend these schools will solely be focusing on their nursing educations while they are in school. Students who attend a nursing college or school do have the opportunity to become a midwife or a public health nurse. They have to go through a training institute for their desired field after graduating from the nursing school or college. Japanese nurses never have to renew their licenses. Once they have passed their exam, they have their license for life.

Today

Like the United States, Japan is in need of more nurses. The driving force behind this need this is the fact that country is aging and needs more medical care for its people. The country needs a rapid increase of nurses however things do not seem to be turning around. Some of the reasons that there is a shortage are poor working conditions, an increase in the number of hospital beds, the low social status of nurses, and the cultural idea that married women quit their jobs for family responsibilities. On average, Japanese nurses will make around 280,000 yen a month, which is one of the higher paying jobs. however, physicians make twice the amount that nurses do in a year. Similar to other cultures, the Japanese people view nurses as subservient to physicians. They are considered lesser and oftentimes negative connotations are associated with nurses. According to the American Nurses Association article on Japan, "nursing work has been described using negative terminology such as 'hard, dirty, dangerous, low salary, few holidays, minimal chance of marriage and family, and poor image'".

Some nurses in Japan are trying to be advocates. They are promoting better nursing education as well as promoting the care of the elderly. There are some organizations that unite Japanese nurses like the Japanese Nursing Association (JNA). The JNA is not to be confused with a union, it is simply a professional organization for the nurses. Members of the JNA lobby politicians and produces publications about nursing. According to the American Nurses Association's article on Japan the JNA, "works toward the improvement in nursing practice through many activities including the development of a policy research group to influence policy development, a code of ethics for nurses, and standards of nursing practice". The JNA also provides certification for specialists in mental health, oncology and community health. The JNA is not the only nursing organization in Japan. There are other subgroups that are typically categorized by the nurses' specialty, like emergency nursing or disaster nursing. One of the older unions that relates to nursing is the Japanese Federation of Medical Workers Union, which was created in 1957. It is a union that includes physicians as well as nurses. This organization was involved with the Nursing Human Resource Law.

Taiwan

- In Taiwan, the Ministry of Health and Welfare is in charge of the regulation of nursing. The Taiwan Union of Nurses Association (TUNA) is the union unit in Taiwan, fighting for nurses on payment and working time issues.

United States

In the US, scope of practice is determined by the state or territory in which a nurse is licensed. Each state has its own laws, rules, and regulations governing nursing care. Usually the making of such rules and regulations is delegated to a state board of nursing, which performs day-to-day administration of these rules, licenses nurses and nursing assistants, and makes decisions on nursing issues. In some states, the terms "nurse" or "nursing" may only be used in conjunction with the practice of a registered nurse (RN) or licensed practical or vocational nurse (LPN/LVN).

In the hospital setting, registered nurses often delegate tasks to LPNs and unlicensed assistive personnel.

RNs are not limited to employment as bedside nurses. They are employed by physicians, attorneys, insurance companies, governmental agencies, community/public health agencies, private industry, school districts, ambulatory surgery centers, among others. Some registered nurses are independent consultants who work for themselves, while others work for large manufacturers or chemical companies. Research nurses conduct or assist in the conduct of research or evaluation (outcome and process) in many areas such as biology, psychology, human development, and health care systems.

Many employers offer flexible work schedules, child care, educational benefits, and bonuses. About 21 percent of registered nurses are union members or covered by union contract.

Nursing is the nation's largest health care profession, with more than 3.1 million registered nurses nationwide. Of all licensed RNs, 2.6 million or 84.8% are employed in nursing. Nurses comprise the largest single component of hospital staff, are the primary providers of hospital patient care, and deliver most of the nation's long-term care. The primary pathway to professional nursing, as compared to technical-level practice, is the four-year Bachelor of Science in Nursing (BSN) degree. Registered nurses are prepared either through a BSN program; a three-year associate degree in nursing; or a three-year hospital training program, receiving a hospital diploma. All take the same state licensing exam. (The number of diploma programs has declined steadily—to less than 10 percent of all basic RN education programs—as nursing education has shifted from hospital-operated instruction into the college and university system.)

Educational and Licensure Requirements

Diploma in Nursing

The oldest method of nursing education is the hospital-based diploma program, which lasts approximately three years. Students take between 30 and 60 credit hours in anatomy, physiology, microbiology, nutrition, chemistry, and other subjects at a college or university, then move on to intensive nursing classes. Until 1996, most RNs in the US were initially educated in nursing by diploma programs. According to the Health Services Resources Administration's 2000 Survey of Nurses only six percent of nurses who graduated from nursing programs in the United States received their education at a Diploma School of Nursing.

Associate Degree in Nursing

The most common initial nursing education is a two-year Associate Degree in Nursing (Associate of Applied Science in Nursing, Associate of Science in Nursing, Associate Degree in Nursing), a two-year college degree referred to as an ADN. Some four-year colleges and universities also offer the ADN. Associate degree nursing programs have prerequisite and corequisite courses (which may include English, Math and Human Anatomy and Physiology) and ultimately stretch out the degree-acquiring process to about three years or greater.

Bachelor of Science in Nursing

The third method is to obtain a Bachelor of Science in Nursing (BSN), a four-year degree that also prepares nurses for graduate-level education. For the first two years in a BSN program, students usually obtain general education requirements and spend the remaining time in nursing courses. In some new programs the first two years can be substituted for an active LPN license along with the required general studies. Advocates for the ADN and diploma programs state that such programs have an on the job training approach to educating students, while the BSN is an academic degree that emphasizes research and nursing theory. Some states require a specific amount of clinical experience that is the same for both BSN and ADN students. A BSN degree qualifies its holder for administrative, research, consulting and teaching positions that would not usually be available to those with an ADN, but is not necessary for most patient care functions. Nursing schools may be accredited by either the Accreditation Commission for Education in Nursing (ACEN) or the Commission on Collegiate Nursing Education (CCNE).

Graduate Education

Advanced education in nursing is done at the master's and doctoral levels. It prepares the graduate for specialization as an advanced practice registered nurse (APRN) or for advanced roles in leadership, management, or education. The clinical nurse leader (CNL) is an advanced generalist who focuses on the improvement of quality and safety outcomes for patients or patient populations from an administrative and staff management focus. Doctoral programs in nursing prepare the student for work in nursing education, health care administration, clinical research, or advanced clinical practice. Most programs confer the PhD in nursing and Doctor of Nursing Practice (DNP).

Advanced practice registered nurse (APRN)

Areas of advanced nursing practice include that of a nurse practitioner (NP), a certified nurse midwife (CNM), a certified registered nurse anesthetist (CRNA), or a clinical nurse specialist (CNS). Nurse practitioners and CNSs work assessing, diagnosing and treating patients in fields as diverse as family practice, women's health care, emergency nursing, acute/critical care, psychiatry, geriatrics, or pediatrics, additionally, a CNS usually works for a facility to improve patient care, do research, or as a staff educator.

Licensure Examination

Completion of any one of these three educational routes allows a graduate nurse to take the NCLEX-RN, the test for licensure as a registered nurse, and is accepted by every state as an adequate indicator of minimum competency for a new graduate. However, controversy exists over the appropriate entry-level preparation of RNs. Some professional organizations believe the BSN should be the sole method of RN preparation and ADN graduates should be licensed as "technical nurses" to work under the supervision of BSN graduates. Others feel the on-the-job experiences of diploma and ADN graduates makes up for any deficiency in theoretical preparation.

Shortage in the United States

RNs are the largest group of health care workers in the United States, with about 2.7 million employed in 2011. It has been reported that the number of new graduates and foreign-trained nurses is insufficient to meet the demand for registered nurses; this is often referred to as the nursing shortage and is expected to increase for the foreseeable future. There are data to support the idea that the nursing shortage is a voluntary shortage. In other words, nurses are leaving nursing of their own volition. In 2006 it was estimated that approximately 1.8 million nurses chose not to work as a nurse. The Bureau of Labor Statistics reported that 296,900 healthcare jobs were created in 2011. RNs make up the majority of the healthcare work force, therefore these positions will be filled primarily by nurses. The BLS also states that by 2020, there will be 1.2 million nursing job openings due to an increase in the workforce, and replacements. (Rosseter, 2012).

Causes

The International Council Of Nursing (ICN), the largest international health professional organization in the world, recognizes the shortage of nurses as a growing crisis in the world. This shortage impacts the healthcare of everyone worldwide. One of the many reasons is that nurses who pursue to become nurses do so very late in their lives. This leads to a non-lengthy employment time. A national survey prepared by the Federation of Nurses and Health Professionals in 2001 found that one in five nurses plans to leave the profession within five years because of unsatisfactory working conditions, including low pay, severe under staffing, high stress, physical demands, mandatory overtime, and irregular hours. Approximately 29.8 percent of all nursing jobs are found in hospitals. However, because of administrative cost cutting, increased nurse's workload, and rapid growth of outpatient services, hospital nursing jobs will experience slower than average growth. Employment in home care and nursing homes is expected to grow rapidly. Though more people are living well into their 80s and 90s, many need the kind of long-term care available at a nursing home. Many nurses will also be needed to help staff the growing number of out-patient facilities, such as HMOs, group medical practices, and ambulatory surgery centers. Nursing specialties will be in great demand. There are, in addition, many part-time employment possibilities.

Levsey, Campbell, and Green voiced their concern about the shortage of nurses, citing Fang, Wilsey-Wisniewski, & Bednash, 2006 who state that over 40,000 qualified nursing applicants were turned away in the 2005-2006 academic year from baccalaureate nursing programs due to a lack of masters and doctoral qualified faculty, and that this number was increased over 9,000 from 32,000 qualified but rejected students from just two years earlier. Several strategies have been offered to mitigate this shortage including; Federal and private support for experienced nurses to enhance their education, incorporating more hybrid/blended nursing courses, and using simulation in lieu of clinical (hospital) training experiences.

Furthermore, there is a shortage of academically qualified instructors to teach at schools of nursing worldwide. The serious need for educational capacity is not being met, which is the underlying most important preparation resource for the nurses of tomorrow. The decrease in faculty everywhere is due to many factors including decrease in satisfaction with the workforce, poor salaries, and reduction in full-time equivalent. Throughout the span of 6 years the nursing faculty shortage has been written about an increasing amount. Unfortunately, there is no clear consensus or an organized plan on how to fix the ongoing issue.

Continuing Education

With health care knowledge growing steadily, nurses can stay ahead of the curve through continuing education. Continuing education classes and programs enable nurses to provide the best possible care to patients, advance nursing careers, and keep up with Board of Nursing requirements. The American Nurses Association and the American Nursing Credentialing Center are devoted to ensuring nurses have access to quality continuing education offerings. Continuing education classes are calibrated to provide enhanced learning for all levels of nurses. Many States also regulate Continuing Nursing Education. Nursing licensing boards requiring Continuing Nursing Education (CNE) as a condition for licensure, either initial or renewal, accept courses provided by organizations that are accredited by other state licensing boards, by the American Nursing Credentialing Center (ANCC), or by organizations that have been designated as an approver of continuing nursing education by ANCC. There are some exceptions to this rule including the state of California, Florida and Kentucky. National Healthcare Institute has created a list to assist nurses in determining their CNE credit hours requirements. While this list is not all inclusive, it offers details on how to contact nursing licensing boards directly.

Board Certification

Professional nursing organizations, through their certification boards, have voluntary certification exams to demonstrate clinical competency in their particular specialty. Completion of the prerequisite work experience allows an RN to register for an examination, and passage gives an RN permission to use a professional designation after their name. For example, passage of the American Association of Critical-care Nurses specialty exam allows a nurse to use the initials 'CCRN' after his or her name. Other organizations and societies have similar procedures.

The American Nurses Credentialing Center, the credentialing arm of the American Nurses Association, is the largest nursing credentialing organization and administers more than 30 specialty examinations.

Women in Nursing

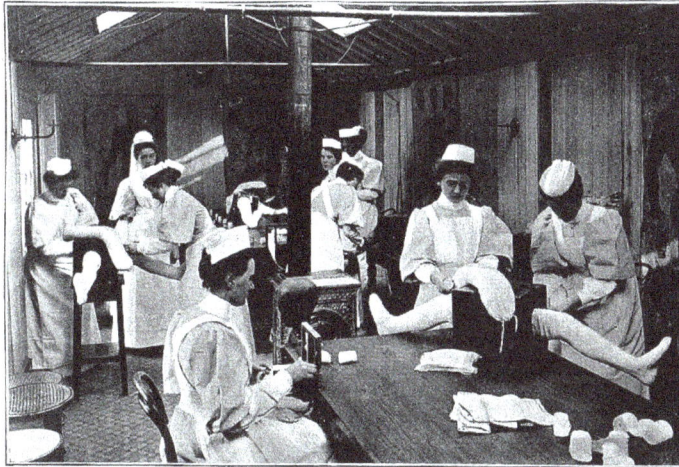

A BANDAGING CLASS AT TREDEGAR HOUSE.
The Preliminary Nurse Training School of the London Hospital.

[*To face p.* 164.

Historically, women have made up a large majority of the profession and academic discipline of nursing. Women's nursing roles include both caring for patients and making sure that the wards and equipment are clean. Currently, females make up the majority of the field of nursing. Statistics show that in 2005, "women comprised 92.3% of Registered Nurses (RNs). Additionally, registered nurses are projected to create the second largest number of new jobs among all occupations between 2004 and 2014, increasing by 29.4%."

Daily Tasks

Nurses in the past were required to work long days and care for many patients, for very little pay. In addition, the typical university setting where nurses learned the work of the trade was not in existence back then. Instead, nurses learned the trade while working in the field. Another difference was that nursing students were called probationers. As probationers, they were required to follow the strict rules and regulations that were set forth by the institution. Additionally, probationers were required to follow all physicians' orders without question and perform various household duties. After learning how to take orders, probationers were then sent to the operating room for a 6-week rotation. During that 6-week period, probationers learned how to inventory sterile bandages, keep operating room meticulously clean and provide sterile water for surgeons during surgery. Upon completion of their training, probationers turned into nurses.

As nurses, some of their roles included providing patient education concerning nutrition and child related illnesses when needed. In general, nurses were the ones responsible for bathing patients, inserting catheters, dispensing medications, administering enemas, keeping the ward clean, and making sure that everything was documented correctly. During that time, there were no nurses' aides available to help with the daily care of patients. Thusly, all tasks fell upon the nurse. To add to that long list of tasks, a nurse was also responsible for preparing any holistic medications that were needed at the time to treat the various alignments that patients presented with. In the present time, holistic medications are hardly used, and any medications that are required are generally handled and prepared by a pharmacy. This is with the expectation of some intravenous (IV), antibiotics, and insulin preparations that the nurse will prepare on the floor (after receiving an order from a doctor). Listed below are more duties of nurses in these time periods.

1880s

- Nurses had 50 patients apiece to care for and were in charge of both their nursing notes and keeping the ward clean. Some of their daily tasks are listed below:

  o Daily sweep and mop the floors of your ward; dust the patients' furniture and window sills.

  o Maintain an even temperature in your ward by bringing in a scuttle of coal for the day's business.

  o Light is important to observe the patient's condition; therefore, each day fill kerosene lamps, clean chimneys, and trim wicks. Wash windows once a week.

  o The nurse's notes are important in aiding the physician's work. Make your pens carefully. You may whittle nibs to your individual taste.

  o Each nurse on day duty will report every day at 7 a.m. and leave at 8 p.m., except on the Sabbath on which day you will be off from noon to 2 p.m.

  o Graduate nurses in good standing with the director of nurses will be given an evening off each week if you go regularly to church.

  o Each nurse should lay aside from each payday a goodly sum of her earnings for her benefits during her declining years, so that she will not become a burden. For example, if you earn $30 a month, you should set aside $15.

  o Any nurse who smokes, uses liquor in any form, gets her hair done at a beauty shop, or frequents dance halls will give the director of nurse's good reason to suspect her worth, intentions, and integrity.

  o The nurse who performs her labors, serves her patients and doctors faithfully and without fault for a period of five years will be given an increase by the hospital administration of 5 cents a day, providing there are no hospital debts that are outstanding.

During the War

- War time saw a demand for nurses. For that demand to be filled, nurses made the transition into the battlefield, leaving their home life behind. On the battlefield, the main duty was to care for the sick and wounded.

After the War

- Completion of the war helped nurses gained a new level of respect from having learned about both anesthesia and psychiatric nursing. Additionally, around this time penicillin was created. This in turn helped to cure many infections and ultimately save many lives.

1950s

- During this generation injections were "still prepared with a pestle and mortar. Oxygen tanks were strapped to beds and there was very little equipment that was disposable. Nurses were in charge of sharpening needles and sterilizing catheter units."

1960s

- The 1960s brought about the development of the Intensive Care Units (ICU) where nurses were required to read telemetry monitors and take patient's blood pressure. In addition to the ICU, the ability to be able to specialize in one field of nursing and obtain an advanced nursing degree (i.e. nurse practitioner degree) become available. Another thing that nurses were required to do (no matter what field they are in) was to stand when doctors entered the room. Lastly, female nurses were still wearing the traditional white uniform and hat.

1970s

- This period saw several changes, with one being that new nurses had to generally work the graveyard shift as they worked their way up in the ranks. Generally, nothing came prepared, which left nurses responsible for mixing, calculating and drawing up both antibiotics and IV medications. To add to this nurses were still using paper charts and medication was kept under lock and key in a cabinet. The last main thing about this period was that nurses were still required to stand when doctors entered the room and the traditional white uniform and hat were still in practice in some facilities but with some modifications.

1980-1990s

- Within this time frame, nurses saw an improvement of technology and its introduction into the field of nursing. The improved technology improved efficiency but it also required that nurses had to go to back to training so that they knew how to use it in practice.

2000s

- Nurses in this period today are still responsible for the direct care of patients (i.e. bathing, feeding, toileting, ambulating, positioning), following doctor's orders, taking vital signs, obtaining daily weights, recording both input and output, obtaining various lab samples, administering medications and charting. It may seem like a lot for one nurse to do in one shift but they are not alone. Meaning that they can delegate some of those tasks to the nursing aide. The ones that they can delegate are the taking of vital signs, recording input and output, obtaining daily weights, and the direct care of patients. There is one important thing that nurses have to think about with delegate though is that they are the ones who are ultimately responsible for the outcomes. To prevent any issues the nurse must first determine if the delegation is within the person's skill level and if the facility allows the nurse to delegate that specific task.

Nurse's Uniforms Throughout History

19th Century

During this time nursing uniforms were very similar to "servants' uniforms, which consisted of a full black or printed gown with a white gathered or banded cap and a white apron." Around 1840, the field of nursing gained more respect and nurses were trained more. With this said the uniforms worn at this time started to change from the servant uniforms to the more classic "lady-like gowns with white aprons and caps to indicate that they were nurses." During this time a very influential nurse started their career in the field of nursing; that nurse was Florence Nightingale. She brought many different things to the field. For instance she helped to make the field a more respectable one with the introduction of both better schooling and uniforms. The improvements in uniforms helped us to determine the rank of all the different nurses practicing. This was accomplished by having nurses wear a hat with a different color band depending on their rank. "Fresh nurse students would wear ribbon bands of pink, blue, or other pastel colors. Senior nurses and nursing teachers would wear black ribbon bands to indicate seniority."

20th Century

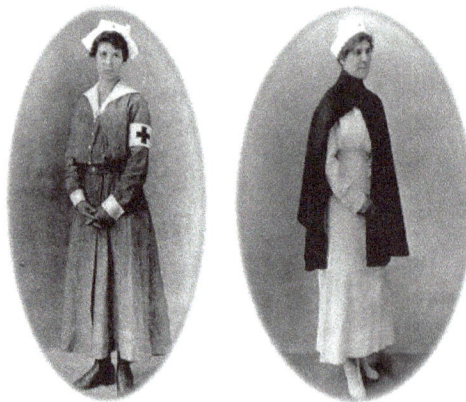

A World War I nurse in a Red Cross ward uniform (left) and another nurse wearing a dark blue cape (right)

This period brought about the start of change in the uniforms by adding white bibs and pockets to the dresses. In addition, large hats were worn that resembled a nun's hat and veil. These types of uniforms stayed in practice up until the First World War, when it was decided that the uniforms needed to be revamped to make them more practical and improve nurses' efficiency. For instance, the sleeves on the uniforms were changed so that they rolled up, the bulky aprons were removed, and the shirts shortened. All these things helped with convenience and allowed nurses to function better, and were often coupled with shoulder-covering capes, which were usually navy or dark blue in colour on the outside with red lining on the inside.

By the 1950s, paper hats and simple folded hats replaced the large, elaborate crown-like caps that were worn by nurses during the First World War. The simple paper hats were more comfortable.

The policy to use hats to denote seniority level was abolished, since the morality of nurses was affected by the discrimination. Dresses also evolved, since no one has the time to launder elaborately tailored clothing anymore. Dresses became less form fitting and were easy to wash, iron and wear."

By the 1970s with the appearance of males in the field wearing scrubs, the female uniforms once again changed, they "became less gendered". The hat was lost and uniforms become less formal. In addition, they started to resemble normal clothing. By the 1980s, the cap and the cloth apron was gone. To replace the cloth apron, nurses started to wear disposable ones.

Today

Nurses today continue to wear scrubs with many different colors and patterns available. The scrubs usually consist of drawn string pants and a V-neck top. The formal uniform (i.e. color and patterns allowed) though varies by policy. In some facilities it is required that the different types of employees all wear different color scrubs so that their specific job title can be determined by their scrub color. For example "nurses in one color, techs in another, etc." Additionally "some hospitals are even going back to requiring that nurses wear white, though they haven't yet returned to skirts, hats, and stockings."

Men in Nursing

Males make up around 20% of the taskforce in the UK and USA. Nurses are typically regarded as female and males in nursing can find themselves referred to by the public and patients as 'male nurses' or 'murse' to distinguish them from other nurses.

History

During plagues that swept through Europe, male nurses were primary caregivers. In the 3rd century, men in the Parabolani created a hospital and provided nursing care. The Codex Theodosianus of 416 (xvi, 2, 42) restricted the enrollment on male nurses in Alexandria to 500.

Reasons for Low Representation

There are several reasons suggested for a low uptake of nursing by males: stereotypes of nursing, lack of male interest in the profession, low pay, nursing job titles such as Sister and Matron, and the perception that male nurses will have difficulty in the workplace carrying out their duties.

Campaigns to Increase Representation

Unlike the campaigns and groups set up to increase and promote women's opportunities in medicine and surgery there have been no comparable campaigns to increase the number of males in nursing.

Whilst there have been no campaigns to increase the number of male nurses in the profession, public perception of men working as nurses is changing, which is seeing larger numbers of men apply for the role.

Careers

Despite there being low numbers of male nurses, there is no indication that they suffer in their career and anecdotal evidence suggests that they can be fast tracked.

United Kingdom

The Society of Registered Male Nurses RCN history merged with the RCN in 1941.

After the Second World War, large numbers of male nurses move into the work force as they were demobilised after the war and had gained medical experience.

In 1951 male nurses joined the main nursing register.

In 2004 the percentage of male nurses was 10.63%. This had increased very slightly to 10.69% in 2008.

In 2008 there were 132 male midwives on the Nursing and Midwifery Council (NMC) nursing register.

United States

In 2008, of the 3,063,163 licensed registered nurses in the United States only 6.6% of were men. Men make up only 13% of all new nursing students.

Nursing schools for men were common in the United States until the early 1900s. More than half of those offering paid nursing services to the ill and injured were men. Yet by 1930, men constituted fewer than 1% of RNs in the United States. As they found other, more lucrative occupations, they left nursing behind.

In 1955, the United States Congress revised the Army-Navy Nurses Act of 1947 to allow for the commissioning of men into military nursing corps.

The American Assembly for Men in Nursing was founded in 1971. The purpose of the AAMN is to provide a framework for nurses as a group to meet, discuss, and influence factors that affect men as nurses.

In *Mississippi University for Women v. Hogan*, 458 U.S. 718 (1982), the U.S. Supreme Court ruled 5–4 that Mississippi University for Women's single sex admissions policy for its nursing school violated the Fourteenth Amendment's equal protection clause. Justice Sandra Day O'Connor wrote the landmark opinion.

Matron

Matron is the job title of a very senior or the chief nurse in several countries, including the United Kingdom, its former colonies, such as India, and also the Republic of Ireland. The chief nurse, in other words the person in charge of nursing in a hospital and the head of the nursing staff, is also known as the Senior Nursing Officer, matron, nursing officer, or clinical nurse manager in UK English; the head nurse or director of nursing in US English, and the nursing superintendent or matron in Indian English, among other countries in the Commonwealth of Nations.

In the United Kingdom, matrons today "have powers over budgets, catering and cleaning as well as being in charge of nurses" and "have the powers to withhold payments from catering and cleaning services if they don't think they are giving the best service to the NHS." Historically, matrons supervised the hospital as a whole but today, they are in-charge for supervising two or three wards.

The chief nurse is a registered nurse who supervises the care of all the patients at a health care facility. The chief nurse is the senior nursing management position in an organization and often holds executive titles like chief nursing officer (CNO), chief nurse executive, or vice-president of nursing. They typically report to the CEO or COO.

History

The word "matron" is derived from the Latin for "mother", via French. The matron was once the most senior nurse in a hospital (in the United Kingdom before ca. 1972). She was responsible for all the nurses and domestic staff, overseeing all patient care, and the efficient running of the hospital, although she almost never had real power over the strategic running of the hospital. Matrons were almost invariably female—male nurses were not at all common, especially in senior positions. They were often seen as fearsome administrators, but were respected by nurses and doctors alike. The National Health Service matron became memorably associated with the formidable character played by actress Hattie Jacques in the 1967 film *Carry On Doctor* and the 1972 film *Carry On Matron*. The matron usually had a very distinctive uniform, with a dark blue dress (although often of a slightly different colour from those worn by her direct subordinates, the sisters) and an elaborate headdress.

Contemporary Matrons

More recently, the British Government announced the return of the matron to the NHS, electing to call this new breed of nurses "modern matrons," in response to various press complaints of dirty, ineffective hospitals with poorly disciplined staff.

They are not intended to have the same level of responsibility as the old matrons, as they often oversee just one department (therefore a hospital may have many matrons—one for surgery, one for medicine, one for geriatrics, one for the accident & emergency department, etc.) but do have budgetary control regarding catering and cleaning contracts. In larger hospitals some will have a group of wards to manage.

Their managerial powers are more limited, and they spend most of their time on administrative work rather than having direct responsibility for patient care.

Many areas of the UK now employ Community Matrons. The role of this staff group is predominantly Clinical and these Matrons have a caseload of patients for whom they are clinically responsible. Many of these patients have chronic health conditions such as COPD, Emphysema, and/or palliative conditions which result in multiple hospital admissions. It is the aim of this staff group to treat the patient within the community thereby limiting hospital admissions. This staff group are predominantly Nurses, but there are other Allied Health Professionals also in the role such as Paramedics and Occupational Therapists.

The nursing branches of the British Armed Forces have never abandoned the term "Matron", and it is used for male as well as female officers, usually holding the rank of Major (or equivalent) or above. It was formerly used as an actual rank in the nursing services.

In South Africa and its former mandated territory South-West Africa (today's Namibia), Matron is the rank of the most senior nurse of a hospital.

Other uses

Long before women were commonly employed as fully sworn police officers, many police forces employed uniformed women with limited powers to search and attend to female prisoners and deal with matters specifically affecting women and children. These female officers were often known as "police matrons". Officers in women's prisons sometimes also used the title of "matron"; sometimes the matron was a senior officer who supervised the other wardresses.

Institutions such as children's homes and workhouses were also run by matrons. The matron of a workhouse was very often the wife of the master and looked after the domestic affairs of the establishment. This was, in fact, the original meaning of the term. Its use in hospitals was borrowed from workhouses.

The term was also used in boarding schools (and is still used in some British independent schools) for the woman in charge of domestic affairs in a boarding house or the school nurse. In the past, the matron was sometimes the wife of the housemaster.

In The Church of Jesus Christ of Latter-day Saints, the female spouse of a temple president or his counselors is referred to as a *temple matron*.

History of Nursing

The word "nurse" originally came from the Latin word "nutrire", meaning to suckle, referring to a wet-nurse; only in the late 16th century did it attain its modern meaning of a person who cares for the infirm.

From the earliest times most cultures produced a stream of nurses dedicated to service on religious principles. Both Christendom and the Muslim World generated a stream of dedicated nurses from their earliest days. In Europe before the foundation of modern nursing, Catholic nuns and the military often provided nursing-like services. It took until the 20th century for nursing to become a secular profession.

Ancient History

The early history of nurses suffers from a lack of source material, but nursing in general has long been an extension of the wet-nurse function of women.

Buddhist Indian ruler (268 B.C.E. to 232 B.C.E.) Ashoka erected a series of pillars, which included an edict ordering hospitals to be built along the routes of travelers, and that they be "well provided with instruments and medicine, consisting of mineral and vegetable drugs, with roots and fruits"; "Whenever there is no provision of drugs, medical roots, and herbs, they are to be supplied, and skilful physicians appointed at the expense of the state to administer them." The system of public hospitals continued until the fall of Buddhism in India ca. 750 C.E.

About 100 B.C.E. the *Charaka Samhita* was written in India, stating that good medical practice requires a patient, physician, nurse, and medicines, with the nurse required to be knowledgeable, skilled at preparing formulations and dosage, sympathetic towards everyone, and clean.

The first known Christian nurse, Phoebe, is mentioned in Romans 16:1. During the early years of the Christian Church (ca. 50 C.E.), St. Paul sent a deaconess named Phoebe to Rome as the first visiting nurse.

From its earliest days, following the edicts of Jesus, Christianity encouraged its devotees to tend the sick. Priests were often also physicians. According to the historian Geoffrey Blainey, while pagan religions seldom offered help to the infirm, the early Christians were willing to nurse the sick and take food to them, notably during the smallpox epidemic of AD 165-180 and the measles outbreak of around AD 250; "In nursing the sick and dying, regardless of religion, the Christians won friends and sympathisers".

Following the First Council of Nicaea in 325 AD, Christianity became the official religion of the Roman Empire, leading to an expansion of the provision of care. Among the earliest were those built ca. 370 by St. Basil the Great, bishop of Caesarea Mazaca in Cappadocia in Asia Minor (modern-day Turkey), by Saint Fabiola in Rome ca. 390, and by the physician-priest Saint Sampson (d. 530) in Constantinople, Called the Basiliad, St. Basil's hospital resembled a city, and included housing for doctors and nurses and separate buildings for various classes of patients. There was a separate section for lepers. Eventually construction of a hospital in every cathedral town was begun.

Christian emphasis on practical charity gave rise to the development of systematic nursing and hospitals after the end of the persecution of the early church. Ancient church leaders like St. Benedict of Nursia (480-547) emphasized medicine as an aid to the provision of hospitality. 12th century Roman Catholic orders like the Dominicans and Carmelites have long lived in religious communities that work for the care of the sick.

Some hospitals maintained libraries and training programs, and doctors compiled their medical and pharmacological studies in manuscripts. Thus in-patient medical care in the sense of what we today consider a hospital, was an invention driven by Christian mercy and Byzantine innovation. Byzantine hospital staff included the Chief Physician (archiatroi), professional nurses (hypourgoi) and orderlies (hyperetai). By the twelfth century, Constantinople had two well-organized hospitals, staffed by doctors who were both male and female. Facilities included systematic treatment procedures and specialized wards for various diseases.

In the early 7th century, Rufaidah bint Sa'ad (also known as Rufaida Al-Aslamia) became what is now described as the first Muslim nurse. A contemporary of Muhammad, she hailed from the Bani Aslam tribe in Medina and learned her medical skills from her father, a traditional healer. After she had lead a group of women to treat injured fighters on the battlefield, Muhammad gave her permission to set up a tent near the Medina mosque to provide treatment and care for the ill and the needy.

Medieval Europe

Medieval hospitals in Europe followed a similar pattern to the Byzantine. They were religious communities, with care provided by monks and nuns. (An old French term for hospital is *hôtel-Dieu*, "hostel of God.") Some were attached to monasteries; others were independent and had their own endowments, usually of property, which provided income for their support. Some hospitals were multi-functional while others were founded for specific purposes such as leper hospitals, or as refuges for the poor, or for pilgrims: not all cared for the sick. The first Spanish hospital, founded by the Catholic Visigoth bishop Masona in 580AD at Mérida, was a *xenodochium* designed as an inn for travellers (mostly pilgrims to the shrine of Eulalia of Mérida) as well as a hospital for citizens and local farmers. The hospital's endowment consisted of farms to feed its patients and guests. From the account given by Paul the Deacon we learn that this hospital was supplied with physicians and nurses, whose mission included the care the sick wherever they were found, "slave or free, Christian or Jew."

During the late 700s and early 800s, Emperor Charlemagne decreed that those hospitals which had been well conducted before his time and had fallen into decay should be restored in accordance with the needs of the time. He further ordered that a hospital should be attached to each cathedral and monastery.

During the tenth century the monasteries became a dominant factor in hospital work. The famous Benedictine Abbey of Cluny, founded in 910, set the example which was widely imitated throughout France and Germany. Besides its infirmary for the religious, each monastery had a hospital in which externs were cared for. These were in charge of the *eleemosynarius*, whose duties, carefully prescribed by the rule, included every sort of service that the visitor or patient could require.

As the eleemosynarius was obliged to seek out the sick and needy in the neighborhood, each monastery became a center for the relief of suffering. Among the monasteries notable in this respect were those of the Benedictines at Corbie in Picardy, Hirschau, Braunweiler, Deutz, Ilsenburg, Liesborn, Pram, and Fulda; those of the Cistercians at Arnsberg, Baumgarten, Eberbach, Himmenrode, Herrnalb, Volkenrode, and Walkenried.

No less efficient was the work done by the diocesan clergy in accordance with the disciplinary enactments of the councils of Aachen (817, 836), which prescribed that a hospital should be maintained in connection with each collegiate church. The canons were obliged to contribute towards the support of the hospital, and one of their number had charge of the inmates. As these hospitals were located in cities, more numerous demands were made upon them than upon those attached to the monasteries. In this movement the bishop naturally took the lead, hence the hospitals founded by Heribert (died 1021) in Cologne, Godard (died 1038) in Hildesheim, Conrad (died 975) in Constance, and Ulrich (died 973) in Augsburg. But similar provision was made by the other churches; thus at Trier the hospitals of St. Maximin, St. Matthew, St. Simeon, and St. James took their names from the churches to which they were attached. During the period 1207–1577 no less than 155 hospitals were founded in Germany.

The Ospedale Maggiore, traditionally named Ca' Granda (i.e. Big House), in Milan, northern Italy, was constructed to house one of the first community hospitals, the largest such undertaking of the fifteenth century. Commissioned by Francesco Sforza in 1456 and designed by Antonio Filarete it is among the first examples of Renaissance architecture in Lombardy.

The Normans brought their hospital system along when they conquered England in 1066. By merging with traditional land-tenure and customs, the new charitable houses became popular and were distinct from both English monasteries and French hospitals. They dispensed alms and some medicine, and were generously endowed by the nobility and gentry who counted on them for spiritual rewards after death.

According to Geoffrey Blainey, the Catholic Church in Europe provided many of the services of a welfare state: "It conducted hospitals for the old and orphanages for the young; hospices for the sick of all ages; places for the lepers; and hostels or inns where pilgrims could buy a cheap bed and meal". It supplied food to the population during famine and distributed food to the poor. This welfare system the church funded through collecting taxes on a large scale and possessing large farmlands and estates.

Roles for Women

Catholic women played large roles in health and healing in medieval and early modern Europe. A life as a nun was a prestigious role; wealthy families provided dowries for their daughters, and these funded the convents, while the nuns provided free nursing care for the poor.

Meanwhile, in Catholic lands such as France, rich families continued to fund convents and monasteries, and enrolled their daughters as nuns who provided free health services to the poor. Nursing was a religious role for the nurse, and there was little call for science.

Middle East

The Eastern Orthodox Church had established many hospitals in the middle east, but following the rise of Islam from the 7th century, Arabic medicine developed in this region, where a number of important advances were made and an Islamic tradition of nursing begun. Arab ideas were later influential in Europe. The famous Knights Hospitaller arose as a group of individuals associated with an Amalfitan hospital in Jerusalem, which was built to provide care for poor, sick or injured Christian pilgrims to the Holy Land. Following the capture of the city by Crusaders, the order became a military as well as infirmarian order.

Roman Catholic orders such as the Franciscans stressed tending the sick, especially during the devastating plagues.

Early Modern Europe

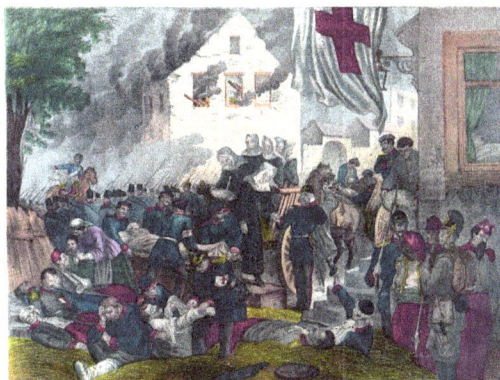

"After the Battle of Gravelotte. The French Sisters of Mercy of St. Borromeo arriving on the battle field to succor the wounded." Unsigned lithograph, 1870 or 1871.

Catholic Europe

The Catholic elites provided hospital services because of their theology of salvation that good works were the route to heaven. The same theology holds strong into the 21st century. In Catholic areas, the tradition of nursing sisters continued uninterrupted. Several orders of nuns provided nursing services in hospitals. A leadership role was taken by the Daughters of Charity of Saint Vincent de Paul, founded in France in 1633. New orders of Catholic nuns expanded the range of activities and reached new areas. For example, in rural Brittany in France, the Daughters of the Holy Spirit, created in 1706, played a central role. New opportunity for nuns as charitable practitioners were created by devout nobles on their own estates. The nuns provided comprehensive care for the sick poor on their patrons' estates, acting not only as nurses, but took on expanded roles as physicians, surgeons, and apothecaries. The French Catholics in New France (Canada) and New Orleans continued these traditions. During the French Revolution, most of the orders of nurses were shut down and there was no organized nursing care to replace them. However the demand for their nursing services remained strong, and after 1800 the sisters reappeared and resumed their work in hospitals and on rural estates. They were tolerated by officials because they had widespread support and were the link between elite physicians and distrustful peasants who needed help.

Protestantism Closes the Hospitals

The Protestant reformers, led by Martin Luther, rejected the notion that rich men could gain God's grace through good works—and thereby escape purgatory—by providing cash endowments to charitable institutions. They also rejected the Catholic idea that the poor patients earned grace and salvation through their suffering. Protestants generally closed all the convents and most of the hospitals, sending women home to become housewives, often against their will.< On the other hand, local officials recognized the public value of hospitals, and some were continued in Protestant lands, but without monks or nuns and in the control of local governments.

In London, the crown allowed two hospitals to continue their charitable work, under nonreligious control of city officials. The convents were all shut down but Harkness finds that women—some of them former nuns—were part of a new system that delivered essential medical services to people outside their family. They were employed by parishes and hospitals, as well as by private families, and provided nursing care as well as some medical, pharmaceutical, and surgical services.

In the 16th century, Protestant reformers shut down the monasteries and convents, though they allowed a few to continue in operation. Those nuns who had been serving as nurses were given pensions or told to get married and stay home. Between 1600 and 1800, Protestant Europe had a few noticeable hospitals, but no regular system of nursing. The weakened public role of women left female practitioners restricted to assisting neighbors and family in an unpaid and unrecognized capacity.

Modern

Modern nursing began in the 19th century in Germany and Britain, and spread worldwide by 1900.

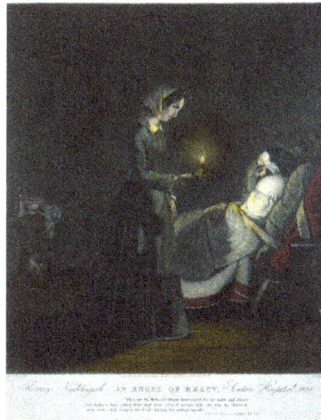

Florence Nightingale, an 'angel of mercy', set up her nursing school in 1860

Deaconess

Phoebe, the nurse mentioned in the New Testament, was a deaconess. The role had virtually died out centuries before, but was revived in Germany in 1836 when Theodor Fliedner and his wife Friederike Münster opened the first deaconess motherhouse in Kaiserswerth on the Rhine. The diaconate was soon brought to England and Scandinavia, Kaiserswerth model. The women obligated themselves for 5 years of service, receiving room, board, uniforms, pocket money, and lifelong care. The uniform was the usual dress of the married woman. There were variations, such as an emphasis on preparing women for marriage through training in nursing, child care, social work and housework. In the Anglican Church, the diaconate was an auxiliary to the pastorate, and there were no mother houses. By 1890 there were over 5,000 deaconesses in Protestant Europe, chiefly Germany Scandinavia and England. In World War II, diaconates in war zones sustained heavy damage. As eastern Europe fell to communism, most diaconates were shut down, and 7000 deaconesses became refugees in West Germany. By 1957, in Germany there were 46,000 deaconesses and 10,000 associates. Other countries reported a total of 14,000 deaconesses, most of them Lutherans. In the United States and Canada 1550 women were counted, half of them in the Methodist Church.

William Passavant in 1849 brought the first four deaconesses to Pittsburgh, after visiting Kaiserswerth. They worked at the Pittsburgh Infirmary (now Passavant Hospital). Between 1880 and 1915, 62 training schools were opened in the United States. The lack of training had weakened Passavant's programs. However recruiting became increasingly difficult after 1910 as women preferred graduate nursing schools or the social work curriculum offered by state universities.

Nightingale's Britain

The Crimean War was a significant development in nursing history when English nurse Florence Nightingale laid the foundations of professional nursing with the principles summarised in the book *Notes on Nursing*. A fund was set up in 1855 by members of the public to raise money for Florence Nightingale and her nurses' work In 1856, £44,039 (equivalent to roughly over £2 million today) was pooled and with this Nightingale decided to use the money to lay the foundations for a training school at St Thomas' Hospital. In 1860, the training for the first batch of nurses began; upon graduation from the school, these nurses used to be called 'Nightingales'.

Nightingale's revelation of the abysmal nursing care afforded soldiers in the Crimean War energized reformers. Queen Victoria in 1860 ordered a hospital to be built to train Army nurses and surgeons, the Royal Victoria Hospital. The hospital opened in 1863 in Netley and admitted and cared for military patients. Beginning in 1866, nurses were formally appointed to Military General Hospitals. The Army Nursing Service (ANS) oversaw the work of the nurses starting in 1881. These military nurses were sent overseas beginning with the First Boer War (often called Zulu War) from 1879 to 1881. They were also dispatched to serve during the Egyptian Campaign in 1882 and the Sudan War of 1883 to 1884. During the Sudan War members of the Army Nursing Service nursed in hospital ships on the Nile as well as the Citadel in Cairo. Almost 2000 nurses served during the second Boer War, the Anglo-Boer War of 1899 to 1902, alongside nurses who were part of the colonial armies of Australia, Canada and New Zealand. They served in tented field hospitals. 23 Army Nursing sisters from Britain lost their lives from disease outbreaks.

New Zealand

New Zealand was the first country to regulate nurses nationally, with adoption of the Nurses Registration Act on the 12 September 1901. It was here in New Zealand that Ellen Dougherty became the first registered nurse.

Canada

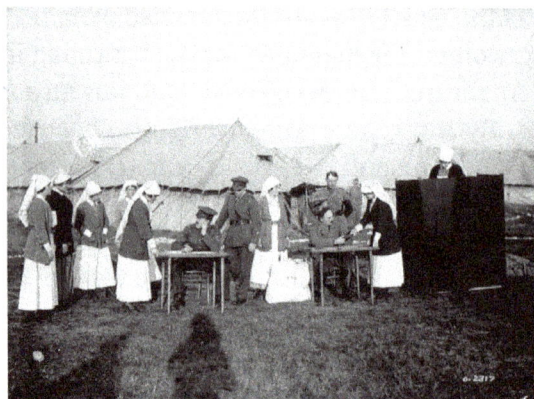

Nursing sisters at a Canadian military hospital in France voting in the Canadian federal election, 1917.

Canadian nursing dates all the way back to 1639 in Quebec with the Augustine nuns.These nuns were trying to open up a mission that cared for the spiritual and physical needs of patients. The establishment of this mission created the first nursing apprenticeship training in North America.

In the nineteenth century there were some Catholic orders of nursing that were trying to spread their message across Canada. These women had only an occasional consultations with a physician. Towards the end of the nineteenth century hospital care and medical services had been improved and expanded. Much of this was due to the Nightingale model, which prevailed in English Canada. In 1874 the first formal nursing training program was started at the General and Marine Hospital in St. Catharines in Ontario. Many programs popped up in hospitals across Canada after this one was established. Graduates and teachers from these programs began to fight for licensing legislation, nursing journals, university training for nurses, and for professional organizations for nurses.

The first instance of Canadian nurses and the military was in 1885 with the Northwest Rebellion. Some nurses came out to aid the wounded. In 1901 Canadian nurses were officially part of the Royal Canadian Army Medical Corps. Georgina Fane Pope and Margaret C. MacDonald were the first nurses officially recognized as military nurses.

In the late nineteenth and early twentieth centuries women made inroads into various professions including teaching, journalism, social work, and public health. These advances included the establishment of a Women's Medical College in Toronto (and in Kingston, Ontario) in 1883, attributed in part to the persistence of Emily Stowe, the first female doctor to practice in Canada. Stowe's daughter, Augusta Stowe-Gullen, became the first woman to graduate from a Canadian medical school.

Apart from a token few, women were outsiders to the male-dominated medical profession. As physicians became better organized, they successfully had laws passed to control the practice of medicine and pharmacy and banning marginal and traditional practitioners. Midwifery—practiced along traditional lines by women—was restricted and practically died out by 1900. Even so, the great majority of childbirths took pace at home until the 1920s, when hospitals became preferred, especially by women who were better educated, more modern, and more trusting in modern medicine.

Prairie Provinces

In the Prairie provinces, the first homesteaders relied on themselves for medical services. Poverty and geographic isolation empowered women to learn and practice medical care with the herbs, roots, and berries that worked for their mothers. They prayed for divine intervention but also practiced supernatural magic that provided as much psychological as physical relief. The reliance on homeopathic remedies continued as trained nurses and doctors and how-to manuals slowly reached the homesteaders in the early 20th century.

After 1900 medicine and especially nursing modernized and became well organized.

The Lethbridge Nursing Mission in Alberta was a representative Canadian voluntary mission. It was founded, independent of the Victorian Order of Nurses, in 1909 by Jessie Turnbull Robinson. A former nurse, Robinson was elected as president of the Lethbridge Relief Society and began district nursing services aimed at poor women and children. The mission was governed by a volunteer board of women directors and began by raising money for its first year of service through charitable donations and payments from the Metropolitan Life Insurance Company. The mission also blended social work with nursing, becoming the dispenser of unemployment relief.

Richardson (1998) examines the social, political, economic, class, and professional factors that contributed to ideological and practical differences between leaders of the Alberta Association of Graduate Nurses (AAGN), established in 1916, and the United Farm Women of Alberta (UFWA), founded in 1915, regarding the promotion and acceptance of midwifery as a recognized subspecialty of registered nurses. Accusing the AAGN of ignoring the medical needs of rural Alberta women, the leaders of the UFWA worked to improve economic and living conditions of women farmers. Irene Parlby, the UFWA's first president, lobbied for the establishment of a provincial Department of Public Health, government-provided hospitals and doctors, and passage of a law to permit nurses to qualify as registered midwives. The AAGN leadership opposed midwife certification, arguing that nursing curricula left no room for midwife study, and thus nurses were not qualified to participate in home births. In 1919 the AAGN compromised with the UFWA, and they worked together for the passage of the Public Health Nurses Act that allowed nurses to serve as midwives in regions without doctors. Thus, Alberta's District Nursing Service, created in 1919 to coordinate the province's women's health resources, resulted chiefly from the organized, persistent political activism of UFWA members and only minimally from the actions of professional nursing groups clearly uninterested in rural Canadians' medical needs.

The Alberta District Nursing Service administered health care in the predominantly rural and impoverished areas of Alberta in the first half of the 20th century. Founded in 1919 to meet maternal and emergency medical needs by the United Farm Women (UFWA), the Nursing Service treated prairie settlers living in primitive areas lacking doctors and hospitals. Nurses provided prenatal care, worked as midwives, performed minor surgery, conducted medical inspections of schoolchildren, and sponsored immunization programs. The post-Second World War discovery of large oil and gas reserves resulted in economic prosperity and the expansion of local medical services. The passage of provincial health and universal hospital insurance in 1957 precipitated the eventual phasing out of the obsolete District Nursing Service in 1976.

Recent Trends

After World War II, the health care system expanded and was nationalized with medicare. Currently there are 260,000 nurses in Canada but they face the same difficulties as most countries, as technology advances and the aging population requires more nursing care.

Mexico

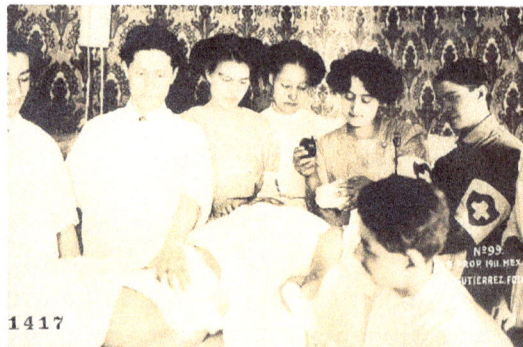

Elena Arizmendi Mejia and volunteers of the Mexican Neutral White Cross, 1911

During most of Mexico's wars in the nineteenth and early twentieth centuries, camp followers known as soldaderas nursed soldiers wounded in warfare. During the Mexican Revolution (1910-1920) care of soldiers in northern Mexico was also undertaken by the Neutral White Cross, founded by Elena Arizmendi Mejia after the Mexican Red Cross refused to treat revolutionary soldiers. The Neutral White Cross treated soldiers regardless of their faction.

France

Professionalization of nursing in France came in the late 19th and early 20th century. In 1870 France's 1,500 hospitals were operated by 11,000 Catholic sisters; by 1911 there were 15,000 nuns representing over 200 religious orders. Government policy after 1900 was to secularize public institutions, and diminish the role the Catholic Church. The lay staff was enlarged from 14,000 1890 to 95,000 in 1911. This political goal came in conflict with the need to maintain better quality of medical care in antiquated facilities. Many doctors, while personally anti-clerical, realized their dependence on the Catholic sisters. Most lay nurses came from peasant or working-class families and were poorly trained. Faced with the long hours and low pay, many soon married and left the field, while the Catholic sisters had renounced marriage and saw nursing as their God-given vocation. New government-operated nursing schools turned out nonreligous nurses who were slated for supervisory roles. During the World War, an outpouring of patriotic volunteers brought large numbers of untrained middle-class women into the military hospitals. They left when the war ended but the long-term effect was to heighten the prestige of nursing. In 1922 the government issued a national diploma for nursing.

United States

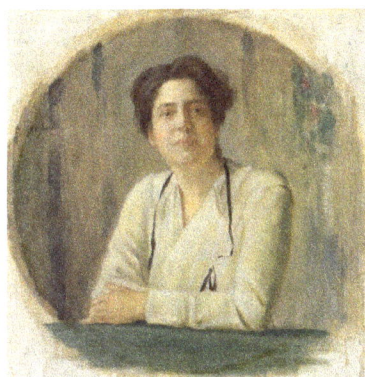

Portrait of Lillian Wald, pioneer of public health nursing, by William Valentine Schevill,
National Portrait Gallery in Washington, D.C.

Nursing professionalized rapidly in the late 19th century as larger hospitals set up nursing schools that attracted ambitious women from middle- and working-class backgrounds. Agnes Elizabeth Jones and Linda Richards established quality nursing schools in the U.S. and Japan; Linda Richards was officially America's first professionally trained nurse, having been trained at Florence Nightingale's training school, and subsequently graduating in 1873 from the *New England Hospital for Women and Children* in Boston

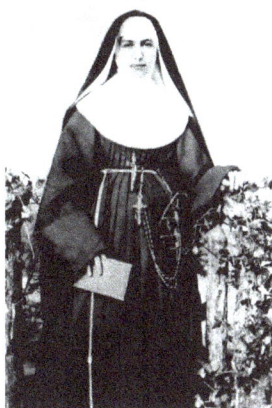

Saint Marianne Cope was among many Catholic nuns to influence the
development of modern hospitals and nursing.

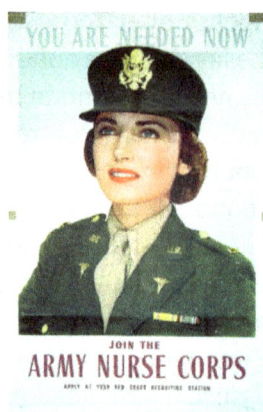

World War II Recruiting poster for the United States Army Nurse Corps (founded 1901)

In the early 1900s, the autonomous, nursing-controlled, Nightingale-era schools came to an end. Despite the establishment of university-affiliated nursing schools, such as Columbia and Yale, hospital training programs were dominant. Formal "book learning" was discouraged in favor of clinical experience through an apprenticeship. In order to meet a growing demand, hospitals used student nurses as cheap labor at the expense of quality formal education.

Hospitals

The number of hospitals grew from 149 in 1873 to 4,400 in 1910 (with 420,000 beds) to 6,300 in 1933, primarily because the public trusted hospitals more and could afford more intensive and professional care.

They were operated by city, state and federal agencies, by churches, by stand-alone non-profits, and by for-profit enterprises run by a local doctor. All the major denominations built hospitals; in 1915, the Catholic Church ran 541, staffed primarily by unpaid nuns. The others sometimes had a small cadre of deaconesses as staff. Most larger hospitals operated a school of nursing, which provided training to young women, who in turn did much of the staffing on an unpaid basis. The number of active graduate nurses rose rapidly from 51,000 in 1910 to 375,000 in 1940 and 700,000 in 1970.

The Protestant churches reentered the health field, especially by setting up orders of women, called deaconesses who dedicated themselves to nursing services.

The modern deaconess movement began in Germany in 1836 when Theodor Fliedner and his wife opened the first deaconess motherhouse in Kaiserswerth on the Rhine. It became a model and within a half century were over 5,000 deaconesses in Europe. The Chursh of England named its first deaconess in 1862. The North London Deaconess Institution trained deaconesses for other dioceses and some served overseas.

William Passavant in 1849 brought the first four deaconesses to Pittsburgh, in the United States, after visiting Kaiserswerth. They worked at the Pittsburgh Infirmary (now Passavant Hospital).

The American Methodists – the largest Protestant denomination—engaged in large-scale missionary activity in Asia and elsewhere in the world, making medical services a priority as early as the 1850s. Methodists in America took note, and began opening their own charitable institutions such as orphanages and old people's homes after 1860. In the 1880s, Methodists began opening hospitals in the United States, which served people of all religious backgrounds beliefs. By 1895 13 hospitals were in operation in major cities. well

In 1884, U.S. Lutherans, particularly John D. Lankenau, brought seven sisters from Germany to run the German Hospital in Philadelphia.

By 1963, the Lutheran Church in America had centers for deaconess work in Philadelphia, Baltimore, and Omaha.

Public Health

In the U.S., the role of public health nurse began in Los Angeles in 1898, by 1924 there were 12,000 public health nurses, half of them in the 100 largest cities. Their average annual salary in larger cities was $1,390. In addition, there were thousands of nurses employed by private agencies handling similar work. Public health nurses supervised health issues in the public and parochial schools, to prenatal and infant care, handled communicable diseases and tuberculosis and dealt with an aerial diseases.

During the Spanish–American War of 1898, medical conditions in the tropical war zone were dangerous, with yellow fever and malaria endemic. The United States government called for women to volunteer as nurses. Thousands did so, but few were professionally trained. Among the latter were 250 Catholic nurses, most of them from the Daughters of Charity of St. Vincent de Paul.

Nursing Schools

Sporadic progress was made on several continents, where medical pioneers established formal nursing schools. But even as late as the 1870s, "women working in North American urban hospitals typically were untrained, working class, and accorded lowly status by both the medical profession they supported and society at large". Nursing had the same status in Great Britain and continental Europe before World War I.

Hospital nursing schools in the United States and Canada took the lead in applying Nightingale's model to their training programmers:

standards of classroom and on-the-job training had risen sharply in the 1880s and 1890s, and along with them the expectation of decorous and professional conduct

In late the 1920s, the women's specialties in health care included 294,000 trained nurses, 150,000 untrained nurses, 47,000 midwives, and 550,000 other hospital workers (most of them women).

In recent decades, professionalization has moved nursing degrees out of RN-oriented hospital schools and into community colleges and universities. Specialization has brought numerous journals to broaden the knowledge base of the profession.

World War I

Britain

By the beginning of World War I, military nursing still had only a small role for women in Britain; 10,500 nurses enrolled in Queen Alexandra's Imperial Military Nursing Service (QAIMNS) and the Princess Mary's Royal Air Force Nursing Service. These services dated to 1902 and 1918, and enjoyed royal sponsorship. There also were Voluntary Aid Detachment (VAD) nurses who had been enrolled by the Red Cross. The ranks that were created for the new nursing services were Matron-in-Chief, Principal Matron, Sister and Staff Nurses. Women joined steadily throughout the War. At the end of 1914, there were 2,223 regular and reserve members of the QAIMNS and when the war ended there were 10,404 trained nurses in the QAIMNS.

Grace McDougall (1887–1963) was the energetic commandant of the First Aid Nursing Yeomanry (FANY), which had formed in 1907 as an auxiliary to the home guard in Britain. McDougall at one point was captured by the Germans but escaped. The British army wanted nothing to do with them so they drove ambulances and ran hospitals and casualty clearing stations for the Belgian and French armies.

Canada

When Canadian nurses volunteered to serve during World War I, they were made commissioned officers by the Royal Canadian Army before being sent overseas, a move that would grant them some authority in the ranks, so that enlisted patients and orderlies would have to comply with their direction. Canada was the first country in the world to grant women this privilege. At the beginning of the War, nurses were not dispatched to the casualty clearing stations near the front lines, where they would be exposed to shell fire. They were initially assigned to hospitals a safe distance away from the front lines. As the war continued, however, nurses were assigned to casualty clearing stations. They were exposed to shelling, and caring for soldiers with "shell shock" and casualties suffering the effects of new weapons such as poisonous gas, as Katherine Wilson-Sammie recollects in *Lights Out! A Canadian Nursing Sister's Tale*. World War I was also the first war in which a clearly marked hospital ship evacuating the wounded was targeted and sunk by an enemy submarine or torpedo boat, an act that had previously been considered unthinkable, but which happened repeatedly. Nurses were among the casualties.

Canadian women volunteering to serve overseas as nurses overwhelmed the army with applications. A total of 3,141 Canadian "nursing sisters" served in the Canadian Army Medical Corps and 2,504 of those served overseas in England, France and the Eastern Mediterranean at Gallipoli, Alexandria and Salonika. By the end of the First World War, 46 Canadian Nursing Sisters had died In addition to these nurses serving overseas with the military, others volunteered and paid their own way over with organizations such as the Canadian Red Cross, the Victorian Order of Nurses, and St. John Ambulance. The sacrifices made by these nurses during the War in fact gave a boost to the women's suffrage movement in many of the countries that fought in the war. The Canadian Army nursing sisters were among the first women in the world to win the right to vote in a federal election; the Military Voters Act of 1917 extended the vote to women in the service such as Nursing Sisters.

Australia

Australian nurses served in the war as part of the Australian General Hospital. Australia established two hospitals at Lemnos and Heliopolis Islands to support the Dardanelles campaign at Gallipoli. Nursing recruitment was sporadic, with some reserve nurses sent with the advance parties to set up the transport ship HMAS *Gascoyne* while others simply fronted to Barracks and were accepted, while still others were expected to pay for their passage in steerage. Australian nurses from this period became known as "grey ghosts" because of their drab uniforms with starched collar and cuffs.

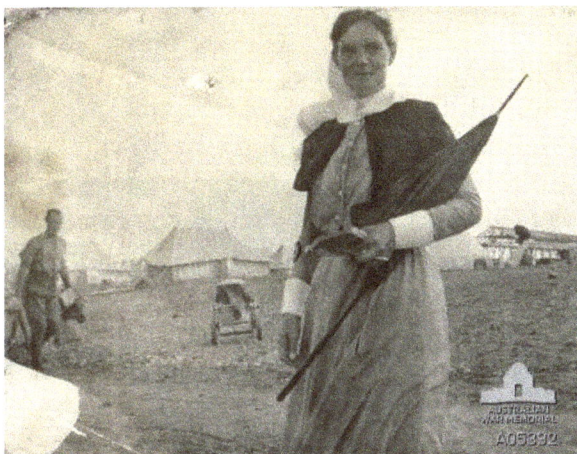

Sister Grace Wilson of the 3rd Australian General Hospital on Lemnos. She sailed from Sydney, New South Wales on board RMS *Mooltan* on 15 May 1915.

During the course of the war, Australian nurses were granted their own administration rather than working under medical officers. Australian Nurses hold the record for the maximum number of triage cases processed by a casualty station in a twenty-four-hour period during the battle of Passchendale. Their work routinely included administering ether during haemostatic surgery and managing and training medical assistants (orderlies).

Some 560 Australian army nurses served in India during the war, where they had to overcome a debilitating climate, outbreaks of disease, insufficient numbers, overwork and hostile British Army officers.

Interwar

Surveys in the U.S. showed that nurses often got married a few years after graduation and quit work; other waited 5 to 10 years for marriage; careerists some never married. By the 1920s increasing numbers of married nurses continued to work. The high turnover meant that advanvcement could be rapid; the average age of a nursing supervisor in a hospital was only 26 years. Wages for private duty nurses were high in the 1920s—$1,300 a year when working full-time in patients' homes or at their private rooms in hospitals. This was more than double what a woman could earn as a teacher or in office work. Rates fell sharply when the Great Depression came in 1929, and continuous work was much harder to find.

World War II

Canada

Over 4000 women served as nurses in uniform in the Canadian Armed Forces during the Second World War. They were called "Nursing Sisters" and had already been professionally trained in civilian life. However, in military service they achieved an elite status well above what they had experienced as civilians. The Nursing Sisters had much more responsibility and autonomy, and had more opportunity to use their expertise, then civilian nurses. They were often close to the front lines, and the military doctors – all men – delegated significant responsibility to the nurses because of the high level of casualties, the shortages of physicians, and extreme working conditions.

Australia

In 1942, sixty five front line nurses from the General Hospital Division in British Singapore were ordered aboard the Vyner Brook and Empire Star for evacuation, rather than caring for wounded. The ships were strafed with machine gun fire by Japanese planes. Sisters Vera Torney and Margaret Anderson were awarded medals when they could find nothing else on the crowded deck and covered their patients with their own bodies. A version of this action was honoured in the film *Paradise Road*. The Vyner Brook was bombed and sank quickly in shallow water of the Sumatra Strait and all but twenty-one were lost at sea, presumed drowned. The remaining nurses swam ashore at Mentok, Sumatra. The twenty-one nurses and some British and Australian troops were marched into the sea and killed with machine gun fire in the Banka Island massacre. Sister Vivian Bullwinkel was the only survivor. She became Australia's premier nursing war hero when she nursed wounded British soldiers in the jungle for three weeks, despite her own flesh wound. She survived on the charity provided by Indonesian locals, but eventually hunger and the privations of hiding in mangrove swamp forced her to surrender. She remained imprisoned for the remainder of the war.

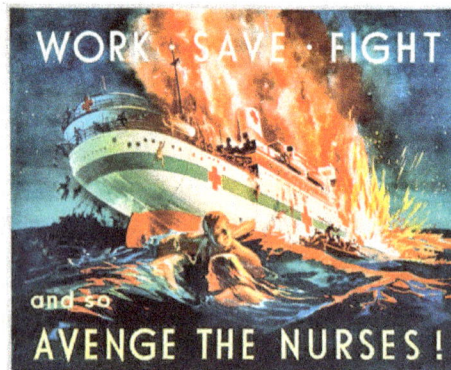

Centaur poster

At around the same time, another group of twelve nurses stationed at the Rabaul mission in New Guinea were captured along with missionaries by invading Japanese troops and interred at their camp for two years. They cared for a number of British, Australian and American wounded. Toward the end of the war, they were transferred to a concentration camp in Kyoto and imprisoned under freezing conditions and forced into hard labour.

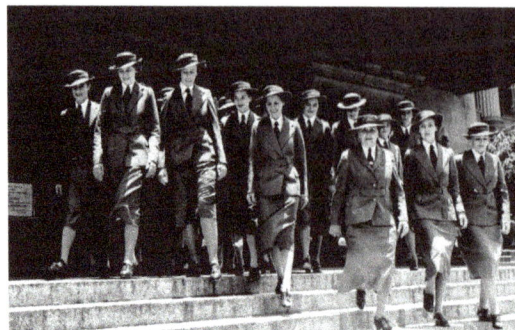

Australian sisters

United States

As Campbell (1984) shows, the nursing profession was transformed by World War Two. Army and Navy nursing was highly attractive and a larger proportion of nurses volunteered for service higher than any other occupation in American society.

The public image of the nurses was highly favorable during the war, as the simplified by such Hollywood films as "Cry 'Havoc'" which made the selfless nurses heroes under enemy fire. Some nurses were captured by the Japanese, but in practice they were kept out of harm's way, with the great majority stationed on the home front. However, 77 were stationed in the jungles of the Pacific, where their uniform consisted of "khaki slacks, mud, shirts, mud, field shoes, mud, and fatigues." The medical services were large operations, with over 600,000 soldiers, and ten enlisted men for every nurse. Nearly all the doctors were men, with women doctors allowed only to examine the WAC.

President Franklin D. Roosevelt hailed the service of nurses in the war effort in his final "Fireside Chat" of January 6, 1945. Expecting heavy casualties in the invasion of Japan, he called for a compulsory draft of nurses. The casualties never happened and there was never a draft of American nurses.

Britain

During World War II, nurses belonged to Queen Alexandra's Imperial Military Nursing Service (QAIMNS), as they had during World War I, and as they remain today. (Nurses belonging to the QAIMNS are informally called "QA"s.) Members of the Army Nursing Service served in every overseas British military campaign during World War II, as well as at military hospitals in Britain. At the beginning of World War II, nurses held officer status with equivalent rank, but were not commissioned officers. In 1941, emergency commissions and a rank structure were created, conforming with the structure used in the rest of the British Army. Nurses were given rank badges and were now able to be promoted to ranks from Lieutenant through to Brigadier. Nurses were exposed to all dangers during the War, and some were captured and became prisoners of war.

Germany

Germany had a very large and well organized nursing service, with three main organizations, one for Catholics, one for Protestants, and the DRK (Red Cross). In 1934 the Nazis set up their own nursing unit, the Brown Nurses, absorbing one of the smaller groups, bringing it up to 40,000 members. It set up kindergartens, hoping to seize control of the minds of the younger Germans, in competition with the other nursing organizations. Civilian psychiatric nurses who were Nazi party members participated in the killings of invalids, although the process was shrouded in euphemisms and denials.

Military nursing was primarily handled by the DRK, which came under partial Nazi control. Front line medical services were provided by male medics and doctors. Red Cross nurses served widely within the military medical services, staffing the hospitals that perforce were close to the front lines and at risk of bombing attacks. Two dozen were awarded the highly prestigious Iron Cross for heroism under fire. They are among the 470,000 German women who served with the military.

References

- Tim McHugh, "Expanding Women's Rural Medical Work in Early Modern Brittany: The Daughters of the Holy Spirit," Journal of the History of Medicine and Allied Sciences (2012) 67#3 pp 428–456. in project MJUSE

- Wilson-Sammie, Katherine M. (1981). Lights Out! A Canadian Nursing Sister's Tale. Mikey. p. 168. ISBN 9780919303515

- Scrubs, Learning About (1 February 2013). "Learning About Scrubs: The History Of Nursing Uniforms". Retrieved 9 April 2015

- Barker, Anne M. (2009). Advanced practice nursing: essential knowledge for the profession. Sudbury, Mass.: Jones and Bartlett Publishers. p. 10-11. ISBN 978-0763748999

- Sasmann, Catherine (7 May 2010). "Kamboi Hulda Shipanga: Namibia's first black matron (1926 to 2010)". New Era. Retrieved 7 May 2010

- Rivett, Geoffery. "NHS History 1948-1967". Archived from the original on 21 August 2006. Retrieved 29 October 2006

- "QAIMNS World War I Queen Alexandra's Imperial Military Nursing Service QAIMNS Nurses". qaranc.co.uk. Retrieved 31 October 2011

2

Nursing Theory and Processes

Nursing theory is the development of techniques and facilities to improve the care of patients. Adaptation model of nursing, Levine's conservation model for nursing, Neuman systems model, self-care deficit nursing theory and Roper–Logan–Tierney model of nursing are some of the theories discussed in the following chapter. This chapter elucidates the crucial theories and principles of nursing.

Nursing Theory

Nursing theory is defined as 'a creative and rigorous structuring of ideas that project a tentative, purposeful, and systematic view of phenomena'. Through systematic inquiry, whether in nursing research or practice, nurses are able to develop knowledge relevant to improving the care of patients. Theory refers to "a coherent group of general propositions used as principles of explanation"

Importance of Nursing Theories

In the early part of nursing's history, there was little formal nursing knowledge. As nursing education developed, the need to categorize knowledge led to development of nursing theory to help nurses evaluate increasingly complex client care situations.

Nursing theories give a plan for reflection in which to examine a certain direction in where the plan needs to head. As new situations are encountered, this framework provides an arrangement for management, investigation and decision-making. Nursing theories also administer a structure for communicating with other nurses and with other representatives and members of the health care team. Nursing theories assist the development of nursing in formulating beliefs, values and goals. They help to define the different particular contribution of nursing with the care of clients. its important for researches, and as a guideline for practical

Types of Nursing Theories

Grand Nursing Theories

Grand nursing theories have the broadest scope and present general concepts and propositions. Theories at this level may both reflect and provide insights useful for practice but are not designed for empirical testing. This limits the use of grand nursing theories for directing, explaining, and predicting nursing in particular situations. Theories at this level are intended to be pertinent to all instances of nursing. Grand theories consist of conceptual frameworks defining broad perspectives for practice and ways of looking at nursing phenomena based on the perspectives.

Mid-range Nursing Theories

Middle-range nursing theories are narrower in scope than grand nursing theories and offer an effective bridge between grand nursing theories and nursing practice. They present concepts and a lower level of abstraction and hold great promise for increasing theory-based research and nursing practice strategies.

Nursing Practice Theories

Nursing practice theories have the most limited scope and level of abstraction and are developed for use within a specific range of nursing situations. Nursing practice theories provide frameworks for nursing interventions, and predict outcomes and the impact of nursing practice.

Nursing Models

Nursing models are usually described as a representation of reality or a more simple way of organising a complex phenomenon. Nursing model is a consolidation of both concepts and the assumption that combine them into a meaningful arrangement. A model is a way of presenting a situation in such a way that it shows the logical terms in order to showcase the structure of the original idea. The term nursing model cannot be used interchangeably with nursing theory both are different.

Components of Nursing Modeling

There are three main key components to a nursing model:

- Statement of goal that the nurse is trying to achieve

- Set of beliefs and values

- Awareness, skills and knowledge the nurse needs to practice.

The first important step in development of ideas about nursing is to establish the body approach essential to nursing, then to analyse the beliefs and values around those.

Common Concepts of Nursing Modeling

There are four common concepts in Nursing Theory that control and regulate practice, these include:

- The person (Patient)

- The environment

- Health

- Nursing (Goals, Roles Functions)

Each theory is regularly defined and described by a Nursing Theorist. The main focal point of nursing out of the four various common concepts is the person (patient).

Major Nursing Theorists and Theories

- Anne Casey: Casey's model of nursing
- Betty Neuman: Neuman systems model
- Boykin & Schoenhofer
- Callista Roy: Adaptation model of nursing
- Carl O. Helvie, Dr.P.H.: Helvie energy theory of nursing and health
- Dorothea Orem: Self-care deficit nursing theory
- Helen Erickson
- Hildegard Peplau: Theory of interpersonal relations
- Ida Jean Orlando (Pelletier)
- Imogene King
- Isabel Hampton Robb
- Katharine Kolcaba
- Katie Eriksson
- Madeleine Leininger
- Katie Love, PhD: Empowered Holistic Nursing Education
- Margaret A. Newman: Health as expanding consciousness theory
- Martha E. Rogers: Science of unitary human beings
- Paterson & Zderad
- Ramona T Mercer: Maternal role attainment theory
- Rosemarie Rizzo-Parse: Human becoming theory
- Virginia Henderson: Henderson's need theory
- Jean Watson, PhD
- Erickson, Tomlin & Swain: Modeling and Role-Modeling
- Moyra Allen: McGill model of nursing
- Nancy Roper, Winifred W. Logan, and Alison J. Tierney: Roper-Logan-Tierney model of nursing
- Phil Barker: Tidal Model
- Michel Nadot: Cultural mediator model (modèle d'intermédiaire culturel)

Purposely omitted from this list is that most famous of all nurses, Florence Nightingale. Nightingale never actually formulated a theory of nursing science but was posthumously accredited with same by others who categorized her personal journaling and communications into a theoretical framework.

Also not included are the many nurses who improved on these theorists' ideas without developing their own theoretical vision.

Adaptation Model of Nursing

In 1976, Sister Callista Roy developed the Adaptation Model of Nursing, a prominent nursing theory. Nursing theories frame, explain or define the practice of nursing. Roy's model sees the individual as a set of interrelated systems (biological, psychological and social). The individual strives to maintain a balance between these systems and the outside world, but there is no absolute level of balance. Individuals strive to live within a unique band in which he or she can cope adequately.

Overview of the Theory

This model comprises the four domain concepts of person, health, environment, and nursing; it also involves a six-step nursing process. Andrews & Roy (1991) state that the person can be a representation of an individual or a group of individuals. Roy's model sees the *person* as "a biopsychosocial being in constant interaction with a changing environment". The person is an open, adaptive system who uses coping skills to deal with stressors. Roy sees the *environment* as "all conditions, circumstances and influences that surround and affect the development and behaviour of the person". Roy describes stressors as stimuli and uses the term *residual stimuli* to describe those stressors whose influence on the person is not clear. Originally, Roy wrote that health and illness are on a continuum with many different states or degrees possible. More recently, she states that health is the process of being and becoming an integrated and whole person. Roy's goal for nursing is "the promotion of adaptation in each of the four modes, thereby contributing to the person's health, quality of life and dying with dignity". These four modes are physiological, self-concept, role function and interdependence.

Roy employs a six-step nursing process: assessment of behaviour; assessment of stimuli; nursing diagnosis; goal setting; intervention and evaluation. In the first step, the person's behaviour in each of the four modes is observed. This behaviour is compared with norms and is deemed either adaptive or ineffective. The second step is concerned with factors that influence behaviour. Stimuli are classified as focal, contextual or residual. The nursing diagnosis is the statement of the ineffective behaviours along with the identification of the probable cause. In the fourth step, goal setting is the focus. Goals need to be realistic and attainable and are set in collaboration with the person. Intervention occurs as the fifth step, and this is when the stimuli are manipulated. It is also called the 'doing phase' . In the final stage, evaluation takes place. The degree of change as evidenced by change in behaviour, is determined. Ineffective behaviours would be reassessed, and the interventions would be revised.

The model had its inception in 1964 when Roy was a graduate student. She was challenged by nursing faculty member Dorothy E. Johnson to develop a conceptual model for nursing practice. Roy's model drew heavily on the work of Harry Helson, a physiologic psychologist. The Roy adaptation model is generally considered a "systems" model; however, it also includes elements of an "interactional" model. The model was developed specifically for the individual client, but it can be adapted to families and to communities (Roy, 1983). Roy states (Clements and Roberts, 1983) that "just as the person as an adaptive system has input, output. and internal processes so too the family can be described from this perspective."

Basic to Roy's model are three concepts: the human being, adaptation, and nursing. The human being is viewed as a biopsychosocial being who is continually interacting with the environment. The human being's goal through this interaction is adaptation. According to Roy and Roberts (1981, p. 43), 'The person has two major internal processing subsystems, the regulator and the cognator." These subsystems are the mechanisms used by human beings to cope with stimuli from the internal and external environment. The regulator mechanism works primarily through the autonomic nervous system and includes endocrine, neural, and perception pathways. This mechanism prepares the individual for coping with environmental stimuli. The cognator mechanism includes emotions, perceptual/information processing, learning, and judgment. The process of perception bridges the two mechanisms (Roy and Roberts, 1981).

Types of Stimuli

- Three types of stimuli influence an individual's ability to cope with the environment. These indude focal stimuli, contextual stimuli, and residual stimuli. Focal stimuli are those that immediately confront the individual in a particular situation. Focal stimuli for a family include individual needs; the level of family adaptation; and changes within the family members, among the members and in the family environment (Roy, 1983). Contextual stimuli are those other stimuli that influence the situation. Residual stimuli include the individual's beliefs or attitudes that may influence the situation. Contextual and residual stimuli for a family system include nurturance, socialization, and support (Roy, 1983). Adaptation occurs when the total stimuli fall within the individual's/family's adaptive capacity, or zone of adaptation. The inputs for a family include all of the stimuli that affect the family as a group. The outputs of the family system are three basic goals: survival, continuity, and growth (Roy, 1983). Roy states (Clements and Roberts, 1983):

- Since adaptation level results from the pooled effect of all other relevant stimuli, the nurse examines the contextual and residual stimuli associated with the focal stimulus to ascertain the zone within which positive family coping can take place and to predict when the given stimulus is outside that zone and will require nursing intervention.

Four Modes of Adaptation

Levine believes that an individual's adaptation occurs in four different modes. This also holds true for families (Hanson, 1984). These include the physiologic mode, the self-concept mode, the role function mode, and the interdependence mode.

The individual's regulator mechanism is involved primarily with the physiologic mode, whereas the cognator mechanism is involved in all four modes (Roy and Roberts, 1981). The family goals correspond to the model's modes of adaptation: survival = physiologic mode; growth = self-concept mode; continuity = role function mode. Transactional patterns fall into the interdependence mode (Clements and Roberts, 1983).

In the physiologic mode, adaptation involves the maintenance of physical integrity. Basic human needs such as nutrition, oxygen, fluids, and temperature regulation are identified with this mode (Fawcett, 1984). In assessing a family, the nurse would ask how the family provides for the physical and survival needs of the family members. A function of the self-concept mode is the need for maintenance of psychic integrity. Perceptions of one's physical and personal self are included in this mode. Families also have concepts of themselves as a family unit. Assessment of the family in this mode would include the amount of understanding provided to the family members, the solidarity of the family, the values of the family, the amount of companionship provided to the members, and the orientation (present or future) of the family (Hanson, 1984).

The need for social integrity is emphasized in the role function mode. When human beings adapt to various role changes that occur throughout a lifetime, they are adapting in this mode. According to Hanson (1984), the family's role can be assessed by observing the communication patterns in the family. Assessment should include how decisions are reached, the roles and communication patterns of the members, how role changes are tolerated, and the effectiveness of communication (Hanson, 1984). For example, when a couple adjusts their lifestyle appropriately following retirement from full-time employment, they are adapting in this mode.

The need for social integrity is also emphasized in the interdependence mode. Interdependence involves maintaining a balance between independence and dependence in one's relationships with others. Dependent behaviors include affection seeking, help seeking, and attention seeking. Independent behaviors include mastery of obstacles and initiative taking. According to Hanson (1984), when assessing this mode in families, the nurse tries to determine how successfully the family lives within a given community. The nurse would assess the interactions of the family with the neighbors and other community groups, the support systems of the family, and the significant others (Hanson, 1984).

The goal of nursing is to promote adaptation of the client during both health and illness in all four of the modes. Actions of the nurse begin with the assessment process, The family is assessed on two levels. First, the nurse makes a judgment with regard to the presence or absence of maladaptation. Then, the nurse focuses the assessment on the stimuli influencing the family's maladaptive behaviors. The nurse may need to manipulate the environment, an element or elements of the client system, or both in order to promote adaptation.

Many nurses, as well as schools of nursing, have adopted the Roy adaptation model as a framework for nursing practice. The model views the client in a holistic manner and contributes significantly to nursing knowledge. The model continues to undergo clarification and development by the author.

Applying Roy's Model to Family Assessment

When using Roy's model as a theoretical framework, the following can serve as a guide for the assessment of families.

- Adaptation Modes

    o Physiologic Mode

- To what extent is the family able to meet the basic survival needs of its members?

- Are any family members having difficulty meeting basic survival needs?

  o Self-Concept Mode

    - How does the family view itself in terms of its ability to meet its goals and to assist its members to achieve their goals? To what extent do they see themselves as self-directed? Other directed?

    - What are the values of the family?

    - Describe the degree of companionship and understanding given to the family members,

  o Role Function Mode

    - Describe the roles assumed by the family members.

    - To what extent are the family roles supportive, in conflict, reflective of role overload?

    - How are family decisions reached?

  o Interdependence Mode

    - To what extent are family members and subsystems within the family allowed to be independent in goal identification and achievement (e.g., adolescents)?

    - To what extent are the members supportive of one another?

    - What are the family's support systems? Significant others?

    - To what extent is the family open to information and assistance from outside the family unit? Willing to assist other families outside the family unit?

    - Describe the interaction patterns of the family In the community.

- Adaptive Mechanisms

  o A. Regulator: Physical status of the family in terms of health? i.e., nutritional state, physical strength, availability of physical resources

  o B. Cognator: Educational level, knowledge base of family, source of decision making, power base, degree of openness in the system to input, ability to process

- Stimuli

  o Focal

    - What are the major concerns of the family at this time?

    - What are the major concerns of the individual members?

  o Contextual

- What elements in the family structure, dynamic, and environment are impinging on the manner and degree to which the family can cope with and adapt to their major concerns (i.e., financial and physical resources, presence or absence of support systems, clinical setting and so on)?

  o Residual

    - What knowledge, skills, beliefs, and values of this family must be considered as the family attempts to adapt (i.e., stage of development, cultural background, spiritual/religious beliefs, goals, expectations)?

The nurse assesses the degree to which the family's actions in each mode are leading to positive coping and adaptation to the focal stimuli. If coping and adaptation are not health promoting, assessment of the types of stimuli and the effectiveness of the regulators provides the basis for the design of nursing interventions to promote adaptation.

Callista Roy maintains there are four main adaptation systems, which she calls modes of adaptation. She calls these the 1. the physiological - physical system 2. the self-concept group identity system 3. the role mastery/function system 4. the interdependency system.

Levine's Conservation Model for Nursing

Myra Levine (a major influence in the nursing profession) set out to find a new and effective method for teaching nursing degree students major concepts and patient care. Levine's goal was to provide individualized and responsive patient care, that was less focused on medical procedures, and more on the individual patient's context. This led to the creation of a new nursing theory and approach to patient care.

The main focus of Levine's Conservation Model is to promote the physical and emotional well being of a patient, by addressing the four areas of conservation she set out. By aiming to address the conservation of energy, structure, and personal and social integrity, Levine's model helps guide nurses in provision of care that will help support the client's health. Though conservation of physical and emotional well being is the most vital part of attaining a successful outcome for patients, two additional concepts, adaptation and wholeness, are also extremely important in a patient's health;

- Adaptation- adaptation consists of how a patient adapts to the realities of their new health situation- the better a patient can adapt to changes in health, the better they are able to respond to treatment and care.

- Wholeness - the concept of wholeness maintains that a nurse must strive to address the client's external and internal environments. This allows the client to be viewed as a whole person, and not just an illness.

- Conservation -the product of adaptation; "Conservation describes the way complex systems are able to continue to function even when severely challenged". Conservation allows individuals to effectively respond to the changes their body faces, while maintaining their uniqueness as a person.

Key Concepts of the Conservation Model

The central concept of Levine's theory is *conservation*. When a person is in a state of conservation, it means that individual has been able to effectively adapt to the health challenges, with the least amount of effort.

Myra Levine described the Four Conservation Principles. These principles focus on conserving an individual's wholeness:

- Conservation of energy: Making sure the client does not expend too much energy, through rest and exercise.

     o *Example: Making sure one's client gets enough sleep and balanced nutrition.*

- Conservation of structural integrity: Doing activities or tasks that will aid in the client's physical healing

     o *Example: Helping the client stay active and promoting good personal care.*

- Conservation of personal integrity: Helping clients maintain uniqueness and individuality

     o *Example: Giving clients choice in how to receive care.*

- Conservation of social integrity: Assisting the patient in maintaining social and community ties will increase their support system during their time in hospital, and will also help the client's sense of self-worth.

     o *Example: Making a pastor available to maintain religious ties during hospitalization.*

Nursing Process Using Levine's Model

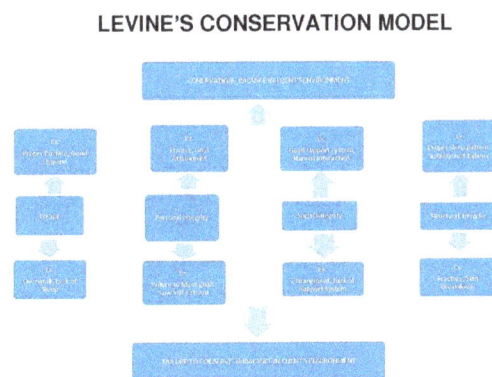

LEVINE'S CONSERVATION MODEL

Levine's Conservation Model Diagram

1. Assessment- The collection of facts, by way of interviews and observation with the patient (considering conservation principles)

2. Judgement (Trophicognosis)- The application of nursing diagnoses which will provide the collected facts with meaning in the context of the patient's circumstance

3. Hypotheses- The application of interventions that aim to maintain the patient's wholeness and promote their adaptation in the current situation

4. Interventions- The use of interventions will test the nurse's hypotheses

5. Evaluation- Assessment of the client's responses to imposed interventions.

Application of the Nursing Process in Levine's Conservation Model

Assessment- The nurse will observe and speak with the patient, in conjunction with medical reports, results and diagnostic studies to gather information- referred to as the collection of *provocative facts.*

Patients will be assessed for challenges to their external and internal environments that may impede their ability to achieve complete wellness and health. Areas focused on which may present such challenges are:

- Energy Conservation- the balance between energy expenditure and the client's energy supply

- Structural Integrity- the defense system for the body

- Personal Integrity- the client's sense of self-worth, independence and validation

- Social Integrity- how well one can be part of a social system (family, community, etc.)

Judgement- Taking the provocative facts of the client's situation and organizing them in a way that makes sense and adds meaning to the patient's circumstances, in order to decide patient needs and possible nursing interventions. Using these judgments to decide about a patient's needs is referred to as *trophicognosis.*

Hypotheses- Using his or her formed judgment, the nurse will speak with the client regarding these judgments with the client. Hypothesizing about the problem and its solution will eventually form a *care plan* for the patient.

Interventions- With the aim of promoting wholeness and adaptation, the nurse tests his/her hypothesis via direct care. These interventions aim to address the four areas of wellness (energy conservation, structural integrity, personal integrity and social integrity).

Evaluation- Evaluation of the interventions aimed at supporting the nurse's hypotheses seek to assess the client's response to the interventions. The evaluation considers both supportive outcomes (providing comfort to the client) and therapeutic outcomes (improving the client's sense of wellness).

Limitations

Due to the fact that Myra's Conventional Model primary focus is on the individual and their wholeness measured by one's personal and emotional well being during a specific period of time, it has been contested that this model is not the best suited when it comes to addressing one's illness in the long term. Thus, the conventions that Myra imposes on nursing students are more driven towards a patient's satisfaction in their current state without looking to future conditions. In addition, satisfying only current conditions does not allow room for nurses to attempt to prevent illness if following this specific model as they are concentrated more on the individual than the illness.

Neuman Systems Model

The Neuman systems model is a nursing theory based on the individual's relationship to stress, the reaction to it, and reconstitution factors that are dynamic in nature. The theory was developed by Betty Neuman, a community health nurse, professor and counselor. The central core of the model consists of energy resources (normal temperature range, genetic structure, response pattern, organ strength or weakness, ego structure, and knowns or commonalities) that are surrounded by several lines of resistance, the normal line of defense, and the flexible line of defense. The lines of resistance represent the internal factors that help the patient defend against a stressor, the normal line of defense represents the person's state of equilibrium, and the flexible line of defense depicts the dynamic nature that can rapidly alter over a short period of time.

The purpose of the nurse is to retain this system's stability through the three levels of prevention:

1. Primary prevention to protect the normal line and strengthen the flexible line of defense.

2. Secondary prevention to strengthen internal lines of resistance, reducing the reaction, and increasing resistance factors.

3. Tertiary prevention to readapt and stabilize and protect reconstitution or return to wellness following treatment.

Self-care Deficit Nursing Theory

The self-care deficit nursing theory is a grand nursing theory that was developed between 1959 and 2001 by Dorothea Orem. The theory is also referred to as the Orem's Model of Nursing. It is particularly used in rehabilitation and primary care settings, where the patient is encouraged to be as independent as possible.

Central Philosophy

The nursing theory is based upon the philosophy that all "patients wish to care for themselves". They can recover more quickly and holistically if they are allowed to perform their own self-cares to the best of their ability.

Self-care Requisites

Self-care requisites are groups of needs or requirements that Orem identified. They are classified as either:

- Universal self-care requisites: those needs that all people have

- Developmental self-care requisites

    o maturational: progress toward higher levels of maturation.

    o situational: prevention of deleterious effects related to development.

- Health deviation requisites: those needs that arise as a result of a patient's condition

Self-care Deficits

When an individual is unable to meet their own self-care requisites, a "self-care deficit" occurs. It is the job of the Registered Nurse to determine these deficits, and define a support modality.

Support Modalities

Nurses are encouraged to rate their patient's dependencies or each of the self-care deficits on the following scale:

- Total Compensation
- Partial Compensation
- Educative/Supportive

Universal Self-Care Requisites (SCRs)

The Universal Self-Care Requisites that are needed for health are:

- Air
- Water
- Food
- Elimination
- Activity and Rest
- Solitude and Social Interaction
- Hazard Prevention
- Promotion of Normality

The nurse is encouraged to assign a support modality to each of the self-care requisites.

Roper–Logan–Tierney Model of Nursing

The Roper, Logan and Tierney model of nursing (originally published in 1980, and subsequently revised in 1985, 1990 and the latest edition in 1998) is a model of nursing care based upon activities of living (ALs). It is extremely prevalent in the United Kingdom, particularly in the public sector. The model is named after the authors – Nancy Roper, Winifred W. Logan and Alison J. Tierney

Introduction

First developed in 1980, this model is based upon work by Nancy Roper in 1976. It is the most widely used nursing model in the United Kingdom. The model is based loosely upon the activities of daily living that evolved from the work of Virginia Henderson in 1966. The latest book edited by these women 2001 is their culminating and completing work, in which they upgrade their model based on their view of societal needs. The original purpose of the model was to be an assessment used throughout the patient's care, but it has become the norm in UK nursing to use it only as a checklist on admission. It is often used to assess how a patient's life has changed due to illness or admission to hospital rather than as a way of planning for increased independence and quality of life.

Activities of Living

Activities of Living (AL), is to promote maximum independence, through complete assessment leading to interventions that further support independence in areas that may prove difficult or impossible for the individual on their own.

The activities of living assesses the individual's relative independence and potential for independence on a continuum ranging from complete dependence to complete independence in order to determine what interventions will lead to increased independence as well as what ongoing support is or will be required to compensate for dependency. Its application requires that it be used throughout the engagement with the patient (not only on admission) as an approach to problems and their resolution, and as a tool to determine how the patient can be supported to learn about, cope with, adjust and improve their own health and challenges.

The ALs themselves are frequently misunderstood or are assumed to have limited scope, leading to dissatisfaction with the model, when one fails to recognise that the ALs are more complex than the title would lead one to believe. For this reason, it is not recommended in the model that it be used as a checklist, but rather as Roper states "As a cognitive approach to the assessment and care of the patient, not on paper as a list of boxes, but in the nurse's approach to and organisation of their care" and that nurses in clinical practice deepen their knowledge and understanding of the model and its application; it is essential that those using such a widespread tool be competent in its correct application.

The ALs are listed as:

- Maintaining a safe environment
- Communication
- Breathing
- Eating and drinking
- Elimination
- Washing and dressing
- Controlling temperature
- Mobilisation
- Working and playing

- Expressing sexuality

- Sleeping

- Death and dying

These activities, outlining both the norm for the patient as well as any changes that may have resulted from current changes in condition, are assessed on admission onto a ward or service, and are reviewed as the patient progresses and as the care plan evolves. To provide effective care, all of the patient's needs (which are determined by assessing the patient's specific abilities and preferences relative to each activity, based on the factors listed) must be met as practicably as possible through supporting the patient to meet those needs independently or by providing the care directly, most preferably by a combination of the two.

By considering changes in the dependence-independence continuum, one can see how the patient is either improving or failing to improve, providing evidence either for or against the current care plan and giving guidance as to the level of care the patient does or may require. This value only results when the assessment is done frequently as changes occur and if it is combined with health improvement and health promotion. It is not effective in a paternalistic environment where all care is provided for an individual even when self care is possible.

Factors Influencing Activities of Living

The following factors that affect ALs are identified. Nancy Roper, when interviewed by members of the Royal College of Nursing's (RCN) Association of Nursing Students at RCN Congress in 2002 in Harrogate stated that the greatest disappointment she held for the use of the model in the UK was the lack of application of the five factors listed below, citing that these are the factors which make the model holistic, and that failure to consider these factors means that the resulting assessment is both incomplete and flawed. She implored students to support the use of the model through promoting an understanding of these factors as an element of the model.

These factors do not stand alone; they are used to determine the individual's relative independence (and requirements to restore independence) for each other activities of daily living.

- Biological- the impact of overall health, of current illness or injury, and the scope of the individual's anatomy and physiology all are considered under this aspect. An example is how having diabetes mellitus causes the person's nutritional activities to differ from those of a person without diabetes.

- Psychological- the impact of not only emotion, but cognition, spiritual beliefs and the ability to understand. Roper explained this was about "knowing, thinking, hoping, feeling and believing". One example of the application of this factor would be how having paranoid thoughts might influence independence in communication; another example would be how lack of literacy could impact independence in health promotion.

- Sociocultural- the impact of society and culture experienced by the individual. Expectations and values based on (perceived or actual) social class or status, or related to the individual's perceived or actual health or ability to carry our activities of daily living. Culture within this factor relates to the beliefs, expectations and values held by the individual both for themselves and by others pertaining to their independence in and ability to carry out activities of daily living. One example is when caring for an individual of advanced age and how societies expectations and assumptions about infirmity and cognitive decline, even if not present in the individual, could influence the delivery of care and level of independence permitted by those with sufficient authority to curtail it.

- Environmental- Roper stated in the interview above that this consideration made hers the first truly "green" model, as it recommends consideration of not only the impact of the environment on the activities of daily living, but also the impact of the individual's ALs on the environment. One example of the environment impacting ALs is to consider if damp is present in one's home how that might impact independence in breathing (as damp can be related to breathing impairments); another example, using the "green" application, would be how dressings that are soiled with potentially hazardous fluids should be disposed of after removal.

- Politicoeconomic – this is the impact of government, politics and the economy on ALs. Issues such as funding, government policies and programmes, state of war or violent conflict, availability and access to benefits, political reforms and government targets, interest rates and availability of fundings (both public and private) all are considered under this factor. One example is how becoming eligible for housing benefit might impact a person's independence, especially if the current housing is poor or inadequate; another example is how living in a place where violence and conflict are the norm would impact the ability to self care.

The Life Span Continuum

The model also incorporates a life span continuum, where the individual passes from fully dependent at birth, to fully independent in the midlife, and returns to fully dependent in their old age/ after death. Some researchers argue that the lifespan continuum begins at conception, others that it begins at birth.

Modifications

Within short-stay settings such as surgery or in areas where the assessor is uncomfortable with or unsure of the applicability of certain activities of daily living (ADL) it is common for the activities 'sexuality' and 'death' (as well as others) to be disregarded. These modifications depend upon the institution or the nurse and often results from a lack of understanding of the application of, or the factors within, the model. This is unfortunate, because this limits the application of the model and thereby reduces its efficacy.

Often clinical settings use a list of the activities of daily living as an assessment document, without any reference to the other elements of the model; Roper herself rejected the use of the list of ADLs as a "checklist" as she stated that it was essential not simply to read the title of the ADL, but to base assessment on knowledge of the scope of the ADL as assessed using the 5 key factors. Roper stated that if nurses themselves were uncomfortable discussing certain factors, they might assume patients also would be and thereby attribute the lack of assessment to the patient's preference, when the patient's opinion was never actually sought.

Roper's assertion leads one to believe that rather than delete or disregard activities of daily living, it can benefit the individual being assessed if the nurse uses the model more thoroughly and assesses the ADL fully, using the 5 factors, irrespective of the area in which the care is being received. Roper stated "The patient is the patient, they are not a different patient because they are in a different clinical area. Their needs are the same- it's who will meet those needs that changes". For example, "sexuality" as an activity of daily living refers not only to the act of reproduction, but also to body image, self-esteem and gender-related beliefs, roles, values and practices, all issues that could have a high degree of relevance for the individual about to undergo surgery. Another example is the ADL "death" which does not only apply strictly to the specific last moments of life, but also to the processes perceived to lead up to the eventuality of death, such as loss of independence, periods of ill health, fear of failure to recover, and fear of the unknown. These are all immeasurably relevant to most or all episodes of care.

Nursing Process

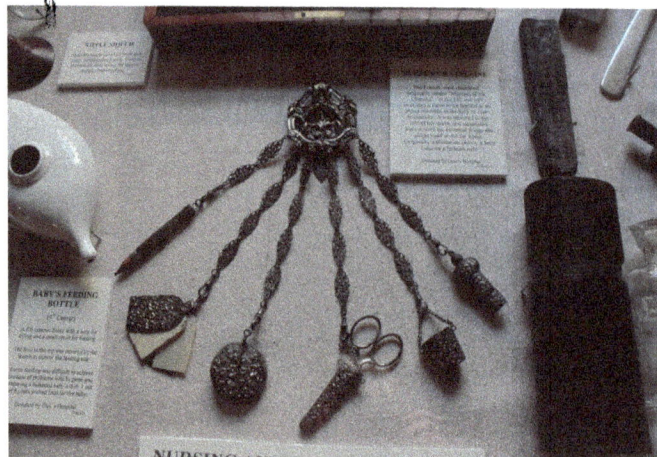

BLW Nurse's Chatelaine or tool kit

The nursing process is a modified scientific method. Nursing practise was first described as a four-stage nursing process by Ida Jean Orlando in 1958. It should not be confused with nursing theories or Health informatics. The diagnosis phase was added later.

The nursing process uses clinical judgement to strike a balance of epistemology between personal interpretation and research evidence in which critical thinking may play a part to categorize the clients issue and course of action. Nursing offers diverse patterns of knowing. Nursing knowledge has embraced pluralism since the 1970s.

Some authors refer to a mind map or abductive reasoning as a potential alternative strategy for organizing care. Intuition plays a part for experienced nurses.

Phases

The nursing process is goal-oriented method of caring that provides a framework to nursing care. It involves six major steps:

- A-Assess (what data is collected?)

- D- Diagnose (what is the problem?)

- O- Outcome Identification - (Was originally a part of the Planning phase, but has recently been added as a new step in the complete process).

- P- Plan (how to manage the problem)

- I- Implement (putting plan into action)

- R- Rationale (Scientific reason of the implementations)

- E- Evaluate (did the plan work?)

According to some theorists, this six-steps description of the nursing process is outdated and misrepresents nursing as linear and atomic.

Assessing Phase

The nurse completes an holistic nursing assessment of the needs of the individual/family/community, regardless of the reason for the encounter. The nurse collects subjective data and objective data using a nursing framework, such as Marjory Gordon's functional health patterns.

Models for Data Collection

Nursing assessments provide the starting point for determining nursing diagnoses. It is vital that a recognized nursing assessment framework is used in practice to identify the patient's* problems, risks and outcomes for enhancing health. The use of an evidence-based nursing framework such as Gordon's Functional Health Pattern Assessment should guide assessments that support nurses in determination of NANDA-I nursing diagnoses. For accurate determination of nursing diagnoses, a useful, evidence-based assessment framework is best practice.

Methods

- Client Interview

- Physical Examination

- Obtaining a health history (including dietary data)

- Family history/report

- Diagnostic Data

- Observation

Diagnosing Phase

Nursing diagnoses represent the nurse's clinical judgment about actual or potential health problems/life process occurring with the individual, family, group or community. The accuracy of the nursing diagnosis is validated when a nurse is able to clearly identify and link to the defining characteristics, related factors and/or risk factors found within the patients assessment. Multiple nursing diagnoses may be made for one client.

Planning Phase

In agreement with the client, the nurse addresses each of the problems identified in the diagnosing phase. When there are multiple nursing diagnoses to be addressed, the nurse prioritizes which diagnoses will receive the most attention first according to their severity and potential for causing more serious harm. For each problem a measurable goal/outcome is set. For each goal/outcome, the nurse selects nursing interventions that will help achieve the goal/outcome. A common method of formulating the expected outcomes is to use the evidence-based Nursing Outcomes Classification to allow for the use of standardized language which improves consistency of terminology, definition and outcome measures. The interventions used in the Nursing Interventions Classification again allow for the use of standardized language which improves consistency of terminology, definition and ability to identify nursing activities, which can also be linked to nursing workload and staffing indices. The result of this phase is a nursing care plan..

Implementing Phase

The nurse implements the nursing care plan, performing the determined interventions that were selected to help meet the goals/outcomes that were established. Delegated tasks and the monitoring of them is included here as well.

Activities

- pre assessment of the client-done before just carrying out implementation to determine if it is relevant

- determine need for assistance

- implementation of nursing orders

- delegating and supervising-determines who to carry out what action

Evaluating Phase

The nurse evaluates the progress toward the goals/outcomes identified in the previous phases. If progress towards the goal is slow, or if regression has occurred, the nurse must change the plan of care accordingly. Conversely, if the goal has been achieved then the care can cease. New problems may be identified at this stage, and thus the process will start all over again.

Characteristics

The nursing process is a cyclical and ongoing process that can end at any stage if the problem is solved. The nursing process exists for every problem that the individual/family/community has. The nursing process not only focuses on ways to improve physical needs, but also on social and emotional needs as well.

- Cyclic and dynamic

- Goal directed and client centered

- Interpersonal and collaborative

- Universally applicable

- Systematic

The entire process is recorded or documented in order to inform all members of the health care team.

Variations and Documentation

The PIE method is a system for documenting actions, especially in the field of nursing. The name comes from the acronym *PIE*, meaning Problem, Intervention, Evaluation.

Nursing Assessment

Nursing assessment is the gathering of information about a patient's physiological, psychological, sociological, and spiritual status by a licensed Registered Nurse. Nursing assessment is the first step in the Nursing process. The Nursing assessment can not be delegated to unlicensed personnel. It differs from a medical diagnosis. In some instances, the nursing assessment is very broad in scope and in other cases it may focus on one body system or mental health. Nursing assessment is used to identify current and future patient care needs. It incorporates the recognition of normal versus abnormal body physiology. Prompt recognition of pertinent changes along with the skill of critical thinking allows the nurse to identify and prioritize appropriate interventions. An assessment format may already be in place to be used at specific facilities and in specific circumstances.

The Client Interview

Before assessment can begin the nurse must establish a professional and therapeutic mode of communication. This develops rapport and lays the foundation of a trusting, non-judgemental relationship. This will also assure that the person will be as comfortable as possible when revealing personal information. A common method of initiating therapeutic communication by the nurse is to have the nurse introduce herself or himself. The interview proceeds to asking the client how they wish to be addressed and the general nature of the topics that will be included in the interview.

The therapeutic communication methods of nursing assessment takes into account developmental stage (toddler vs. the elderly), privacy, distractions, age-related impediments to communication such as sensory deficits and language, place, time, non-verbal cues. Therapeutic communication is also facilitated by avoiding the use of medical jargon and instead using common terms used by the patient.

During the first part of the personal interview, the nurse carries out an analysis of the patient needs. In many cases, the client requires a focused assessment rather than a comprehensive nursing assessment of the entire bodily systems. In the focused assessment, the major complaint is assessed. The nurse may employ the use of acronyms performing the assessment:

- OLDCART

    o   Onset of health concern or complaint

    o   Location of pain or other symptoms related to the area of the body involved

    o   Duration of health concern or complaint

    o   Characteristics

    o   Aggravating factors or what makes the concern or complaint worse

    o   Relieving factors or what makes the concern or complaint better

    o   Treatments or what treatments were tried in the past or ongoing

Patient History and Interview

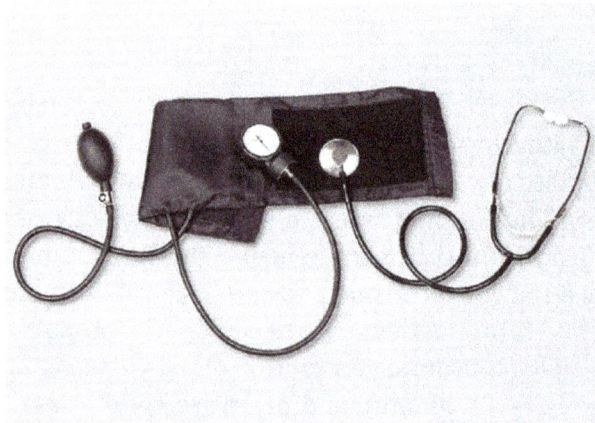

Auscultatory method aneroid sphygmomanometer with stethoscope

The patient history and interview is considered to be subjective but still of high importance when combined with objective measurements. High quality interviewing strategies include the use of open-ended questions. Open-ended questions are those that cannot be answered with a simple "yes" or "no" response. If the person is unable to respond, then family or caregivers will be given the opportunity to answer the questions.

The typical nursing assessment in the clinical setting will be the collection of data about the following:

- present complaint and nature of symptoms

- onset of symptoms

- severity of symptoms

- classifying symptoms as acute or chronic

- health history

- family history

- social history

- current medical and/or nursing management

- understanding of medical and nursing plans

- perception of illness

In addition, the nursing assessment may include reviewing the results of laboratory values such as blood work and urine analysis. Medical records of the client assist to determine the baseline measures related to their health.

In some instances, the nursing assessment will not incorporate the typical patient history and interview if prioritization indicates that immediate action is urgent to preserve the airway, breathing and circulation. This is also known as triage and is used in emergency rooms and medical team disaster response situations. The patient history is documented through a personal interview with the client and/or the client's family. If there is an urgent need for a focused assessment, the most obvious or troubling complaint will be addressed first. This is especially important in the case of extreme pain.

Physical Examination

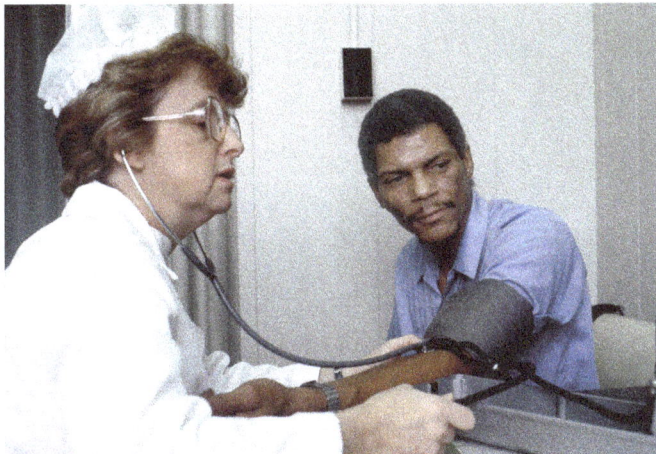

Assessing blood pressure

A nursing assessment includes a physical examination: the observation or measurement of signs, which can be observed or measured, or symptoms such as nausea or vertigo, which can be felt by the patient.

The techniques used may include Inspection, Palpation, Auscultation and Percussion in addition to the "vital signs" of temperature, blood pressure, pulse and respiratory rate, and further examination of the body systems such as the cardiovascular or musculoskeletal systems.

Focused Assessment

Neurovascular Assessment

The nurse conducts a neurovascular assessment to determine sensory and muscular function of the arms and legs in addition to peripheral circulation. The focused neurovascular assessment includes the objective observation of pulses, capillary refill, skin color and temperature, and sensation. During the neurovascular assessment the measures between extremities are compared. A neurovascular assessment is an evaluation of the extremities along with sensory, circulation and motor function.

Mental Status

During the assessment, interactions and functioning are evaluated and documented. Those specific items assessed include:

- orientation, memory,

- mood, depression, anxiety, coherence, hallucinations, illusions, insight

- speech patterns (rate, clarity clanging)

- grooming, personal hygiene, appropriateness of clothing

- response to verbal and tactile stimuli, level of consciousness, and alertness

- posture, gait, appropriateness of movements

Pain

- site, chronicity

Integument

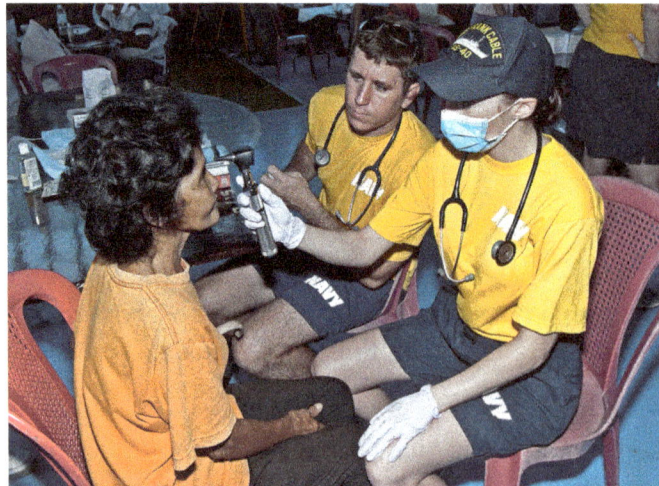
Performing an eye exam by military nurses

- hair: quantity, location, distribution, texture

- nails: shape and color, presence of clubbing

- lesions: type, location, arrangement, color of lesions, drainage, depth, width, length

- texture, moisture, color, elasticity, turgor

Head

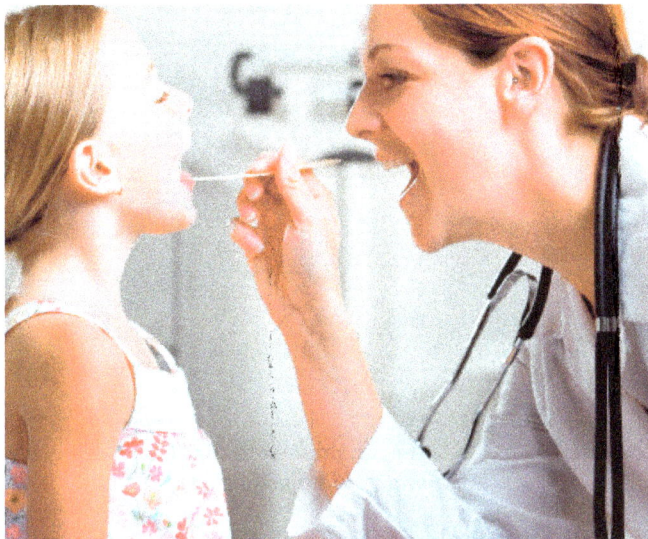

assessing the throat of a child

- scalp, facial symmetry, sensation
- eyes
    - acuity
    - eyelids
    - lacrimal glands
    - conjunctiva
    - visual fields
    - peripheral vision
    - sclera
    - size, shape, symmetry, pupil reactions
    - movement (cranial nerves)
- ears
    - external structure
    - inner ear
    - eardrum
    - hearing (frequencies of sound detected)
- dentation

Psychosocial Assessment

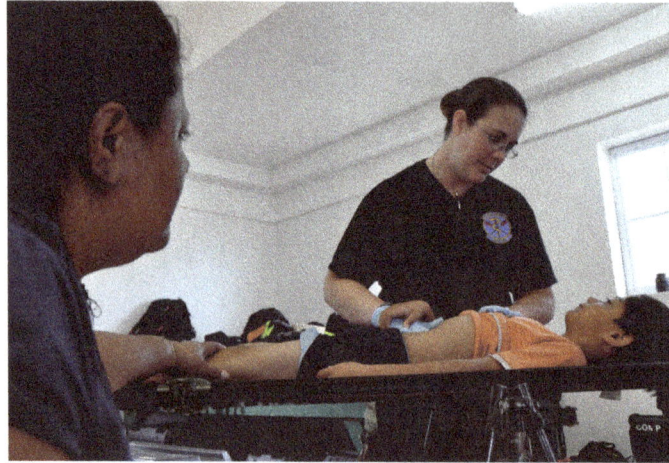
Abdominal palpation of a boy

The main areas considered in a psychological examination are intellectual health and emotional health. Assessment of cognitive function, checking for hallucinations and delusions, measuring concentration levels, and inquiring into the client's hobbies and interests constitute an intellectual health assessment. Emotional health is assessed by observing and inquiring about how the client feels and what he does in response to these feelings. The psychological examination may also include the client's perceptions (why they think they are being assessed or have been referred, what they hope to gain from the meeting). Religion and beliefs are also important areas to consider. The need for a physical health assessment is always included in any psychological examination to rule out structural damage or anomalies.

Safety

- environment

- ambulatory aids

Cultural Assessment

The nursing cultural assessment will identify factors that may impede or facilitate the implementation of a nursing diagnosis. Cultural factors have a major impact on the nursing assessment. Some of the information obtained during the interview include:

- ethnic origin

- primary language

- second language

- the need for an interpreter

- the client's main support system(s)

- family living arrangements

- Who is the major decision maker in the family? What are the family members' roles within the family

- Describe religious beliefs and practices

- Are there any religious requirements/restrictions that place limitations on the client's care?

- Who in the family takes responsibility for health concerns?

- Describe any special health beliefs and practices:

- From whom does family usually seek medical assistance in time of need?

- Describe client's usual emotional/behavioral response to: Anxiety: Anger: Loss/change/failure: Pain: Fear:

- Describe any topics that are particularly sensitive or that the client is unwilling to discuss (because of cultural taboos):

- Describe any activities in which the client is unwilling to participate (because of cultural customs or taboos):

- What are the client's personal feelings regarding touch?

- What are the client's personal feelings regarding eye contact?

- What is the client's personal orientation to time? (past, present, future)

- Describe any particular illnesses to which the client may be bioculturally susceptible (e.g., hypertension and sickle cell anemia in *African Americans):

- Describe any nutritional deficiencies to which the client may be bioculturally susceptible (e.g., lactose intolerance in Native and Asian Americans)

- Are there any foods the client requests or refuses because of cultural beliefs related to this illness (e.g., "hot" and "cold" foods for Latino Americans and Asian Americans)?

Assessment Tools

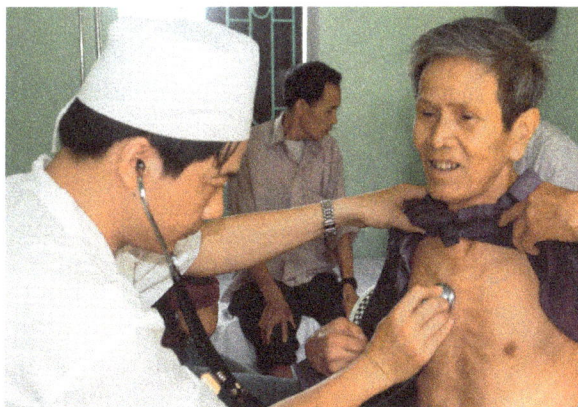

Auscultation assessing lung sounds

A range of instruments and tools have been developed to assist nurses in their assessment role. These include: the index of independence in activities of daily living, the Barthel index, the Crighton Royal behaviour rating scale, the Clifton assessment procedures for the elderly, the general health questionnaire, and the geriatric mental health state schedule.

Other assessment tools may focus on a specific aspect of the patient's care. For example, the Waterlow score and the Braden scale deals with a patient's risk of developing a Pressure ulcer (decubitus ulcer), the Glasgow Coma Scale measures the conscious state of a person, and various pain scales exist to assess the "fifth vital sign"

The use of medical equipment is routinely employed to conduct a nursing assessment. These include, the otoscope, thermometer, stethoscope, penlight, sphygmomanometer, bladder scanner, speculum, and eye charts. Besides the interviewing process, the nursing assessment utilizes certain techniques to collect information such as observation, auscultation, palpation and percussion.

Physical Examination

A physical examination, medical examination, or clinical examination (more popularly known as a check-up) is the process by which a medical professional investigates the body of a patient for signs of disease. It generally follows the taking of the medical history—an account of the symptoms as experienced by the patient. Together with the medical history, the physical examination aids in determining the correct diagnosis and devising the treatment plan. This data then becomes part of the medical record.

A Cochrane Collaboration meta-study found that routine annual physicals did not measurably reduce the risk of illness or death, and conversely, could lead to over-diagnosis and over-treatment. The authors concluded that routine physicals were unlikely to do more good than harm.

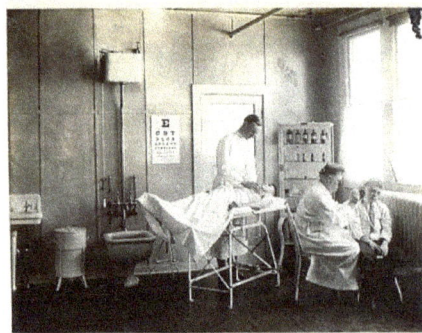

An examination room in Washington, DC, during the first World War

Types

A resident physician at the Granada Relocation Center, examining a patient's throat

Routine Physicals

Routine physicals are physical examinations performed on asymptomatic patients for medical screening purposes. These are normally performed by a pediatrician, family practice physician, physician assistant, a certified nurse practitioner or other primary care provider. This routine physical exam usually includes the HEENT evaluation. Nursing professionals such as Registered Nurse, Licensed Practical Nurses develop a baseline assessment to identify normal versus abnormal findings. These are reported to the primary care provider.

Comprehensive Physicals

Comprehensive physical exams, also known as executive physicals, typically include laboratory tests, chest x-rays, pulmonary function testing, audiograms, full body CAT scanning, EKGs, heart stress tests, vascular age tests, urinalysis, and mammograms or prostate exams depending on gender.

Pre-employment Examinations

Pre-employment examinations are screening tests which judge the suitability of a worker for hire based on the results of their physical examination. This is also called *pre-employment medical clearance*. Many employers believe that by only hiring workers whose physical examination results pass certain exclusionary criteria, their employees collectively will have fewer absences due to sickness, fewer workplace injuries, and less occupational disease.

A small amount of low-quality evidence in medical research supports the idea that pre-employment physical examinations can actually reduce absences, workplace injuries, and occupational disease.

Employers should not routinely request that workers x-ray their lower backs as a condition for getting a job. Reasons for not doing this include the inability of such testing to predict future problems, the radiation exposure to the worker, and the cost of the exam.

Insurance Exams

These are physicals performed as a condition of buying health insurance or life insurance.

Uses

Diagnosis

Physical examinations are performed in most healthcare encounters. For example, a physical examination is performed when a patient visits complains of flu-like symptoms. These diagnostic examinations usually focus on the patient's chief complaint.

Screening

General health checks, including physical examinations performed when the patient reported no health concerns, often include medical screening for common conditions, such as high blood pressure. A Cochrane review found that general health checks did not reduce the risk of death from cancer, heart disease, or any other cause, and could not be proved to affect the patient's likelihood of being admitted to the hospital, becoming disabled, missing work, or needing additional office visits. The study found no effect on the risk of illness, but did find evidence suggesting that patients subject to routine physicals were diagnosed with hypertension and other chronic conditions at a higher rate than those who were not. Its authors noted that studies often failed to consider or report possible harmful outcomes (such as unwarranted anxiety or unnecessary follow-up procedures), and concluded that routine health checks were "unlikely to be beneficial" in regards to lowering cardiovascular and cancer morbidity and mortality.

Establishing Doctor-patient Relationship

In addition to the possibility of identifying signs of illness, it has been described as a ritual that plays a significant role in the doctor-patient relationship that will provide benefits in other medical encounters.

Format and Interpretation

A physical examination may include checking vital signs, including temperature examination, Blood pressure, pulse, and respiratory rate. The healthcare provider uses the senses of sight, hearing, touch, and sometimes smell (e.g., in infection, uremia, diabetic ketoacidosis). Taste has been made redundant by the availability of modern lab tests. Four actions are taught as the basis of physical examination: inspection, palpation (feel), percussion (tap to determine resonance characteristics), and auscultation (listen).

What is Checked

While elective physical exams have become more elaborate, in routine use physical exams have become less complete. This has led to editorials in medical journals about the importance of an adequate physical examination.

Although providers have varying approaches as to the sequence of body parts, a systematic examination generally starts at the head and finishes at the extremities. After the main organ systems have been investigated by inspection, palpation, percussion, and auscultation, specific tests may follow (such as a neurological investigation, orthopedic examination) or specific tests when a particular disease is suspected (e.g. eliciting Trousseau's sign in hypocalcemia).

With the clues obtained during the *history* and *physical examination* the healthcare provider can now formulate a differential diagnosis, a list of potential causes of the symptoms. Specific diagnostic tests (or occasionally empirical therapy) generally confirm the cause, or shed light on other, previously overlooked, causes.

Physicians at Stanford University medical school have introduced a set of 25 key physical examination skills that were felt to be useful.

Example

While the format of examination as listed below is largely as taught and expected of students, a specialist will focus on their particular field and the nature of the problem described by the patient. Hence a cardiologist will not in routine practice undertake neurological parts of the examination other than noting that the patient is able to use all four limbs on entering the consultation room and during the consultation become aware of their hearing, eyesight and speech. Likewise an Orthopaedic surgeon will examine the affected joint, but may only briefly check the heart sounds and chest to ensure that there is not likely to be any contraindication to surgery raised by the anaesthetist. A primary care physician will also generally examine the male genitals but may leave the examination of the female genitalia to a gynecologist.

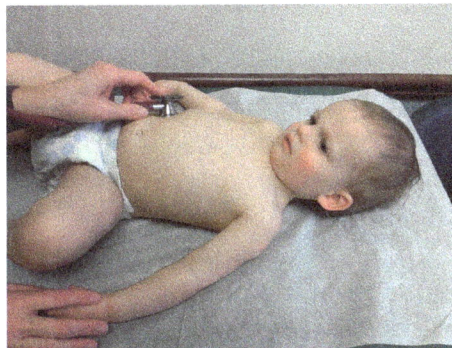

A doctor using a stethoscope to listen to a 15-month-old's abdomen

A complete physical examination includes evaluation of general patient appearance and specific organ systems. It is recorded in the medical record in a standard layout which facilitates others later reading the notes. In practice the vital signs of temperature examination, pulse and blood pressure are usually measured first.

Section	Sample text	Comments
General	"Patient in NAD. VS: WNL"	May be split on two lines. "WNL" = "within normal limits"
HEENT:	"NC/AT. PERRLA, EOMI. No cervical LAD, no thyromegaly, no bruit, no pallor, fundus WNL, oropharynx WNL, tympanic membrane WNL, neck supple"	"Neck" is sometimes split out from "Head". "Good dentition" may be noted.
Resp or "Chest"	"Nontender, CTA bilat" Chest expansion test, normal breathing with little effort, absence of wheezing, rhonchi and crackles.	More detailed examinations can include rales, rhonchi, wheezing ("no r/r/w"), and rubs. Other phrases may include "no cyanosis or clubbing" (if section is labeled "Resp" and not "Chest"), "fremitus WNL", and "no dullnes to percussion".
CV or "Heart"	"+S1, +S2, RRR, no m/r/g"	If "CV" is used instead of "heart", peripheral pulses are sometimes included in this section (otherwise, they may be in the extremities section)
Abd	"Soft, nontender, nondistended, absence of pain, no hepatosplenomegaly, NBS"	If lower back pain is involved, then the "Back" may become a primary section. Costovertebral angle tenderness may be included in the abdominal section if there is no back section. More detailed examinations may report "+psoas sign, +Rovsing's sign, +obturator sign". If tenderness was present, it might be reported as "Direct and rebound RLQ tenderness". "NBS" stands for "normal bowel sounds"; alternatives might include "hypoactive BS" or "hyperactive BS".
Ext	"No clubbing, cyanosis, edema"	Checking the fingers for clubbing and cyanosis is sometimes considered part of the pulmonary exam, because it closely involves oxygenation. Examinations of the knee may involve the McMurray test, Lachman test, and drawer test.
Neuro	"A&Ox3, CN II-XII grossly intact, Sensation intact in all four extremities (dull and sharp), DTR 2+ bilat, Romberg negative, cerebellar reflexes WNL, normal gait"	Sensation may be expanded to include dull, sharp, vibration, temperature, and position sense. A mental status exam may be reported at the beginning of the neurologic exam, or under a distinct "Psych" section.

Depending upon the chief complaint, additional sections may be included. For example, hearing may be evaluated with a specific Weber test and Rinne test, or it may be more briefly addressed in a cranial nerve exam. To give another example, a neurological related complaint might be evaluated with a specific test, such as the Romberg maneuver.

History

The history and physical examination were supremely important to diagnosis before advanced health technology was developed, and even today, despite impressive medical imaging and molecular medical tests, they remain indispensable in many contexts. Before the 19th century, the history and physical examination were nearly the only diagnostic tools the physician had, which explains why tactile skill and ingenious appreciation in the exam were so highly valued in the definition of what made for a good physician. Even as late as 1890, the world had no radiography or fluoroscopy, only early and limited forms of electrophysiologic testing, and no molecular biology as we know it today. Ever since this peak of the importance of the physical examination, reviewers have warned that clinical practice and medical education need to remain vigilant in appreciating the continuing need for physical examination and effectively teaching the skills to perform it; this call is ongoing, as the 21st-century literature shows.

The executive physical format was developed from the 1970s by the Mayo Clinic and is now offered by other health providers, including Johns Hopkins University, EliteHealth and Mount Sinai in New York City. Executive physicals are also the primary service of concierge doctors, who say that they do a more thorough examination for a cash premium on top of the insurance coverage.

Society and Culture

A physical examination may be provided under health insurance cover, required of new insurance customers. This is a part of insurance medicine. In the United States, physicals are also marketed to patients as a one-stop health review, avoiding the inconvenience of attending multiple appointments with different healthcare providers.

Palpation

Palpation is the process of using one's hands to examine the body, especially while perceiving/diagnosing a disease or illness. Usually performed by a health care practitioner, it is the process of feeling an object in or on the body to determine its size, shape, firmness, or location (for example, a veterinarian can feel the stomach of a pregnant animal to ensure good health and successful delivery).

Palpation is an important part of the physical examination; the sense of touch is just as important in this examination as the sense of sight is. Physicians develop great skill in palpating problems below the surface of the body, becoming able to detect things that untrained persons would not. Mastery of anatomy and much practice are required to achieve a high level of skill. The concept of being able to detect or notice subtle tactile signs and to recognize their significance or implications is called appreciating them (just as in general vocabulary one can speak of appreciating the importance of something). Nonetheless, some things are not palpable, which is why additional medical tests, such as medical imaging and laboratory tests, are often needed to make a diagnosis. However, many other problems *are* palpable. Examples include pulses, abdominal distension, cardiac thrills, fremitus, and various hernias, joint dislocations, bone fractures, and tumors, among others.

Uses

Palpation is used by physicians, as well as chiropractors, massage therapists, physical therapists, osteopaths and occupational therapists, to assess the texture of a patient's tissue (such as swelling or muscle tone), to locate the spatial coordinates of particular anatomical landmarks (e.g., to assess range and quality of joint motion), and assess tenderness through tissue deformation (e.g. provoking pain with pressure or stretching). In summary, palpation might be used either to determine painful areas and to qualify pain felt by patients, or to locate three-dimensional coordinates of anatomical landmarks to quantify some aspects of the palpated subject.

Palpation is typically used for thoracic and abdominal examinations, but can also be used to diagnose edema and to measure the pulse. It is used by veterinarians to check animals for pregnancy, and by midwives to determine the position of a fetus.

Quantitative palpation of anatomical landmarks for measurements must occur according to strict protocols if one wishes to achieve reproducible measurements. Palpation protocols are usually based on well-described definitions for the location of anatomical, usually skeletal, landmarks.

Locating Anatomical Landmarks

Locating anatomical landmarks can be performed using two palpation protocols: 1) *manual palpation* that allows spatial location of landmarks using hands combined or not with three-dimensional (3D) digitizing, and 2) *virtual palpation* on 3D computer models obtained, for example, from medical imaging.

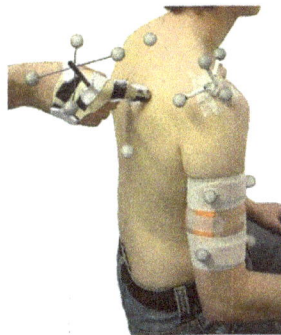

Manual palpation of skeletal landmarks combined with 3D digitizing.

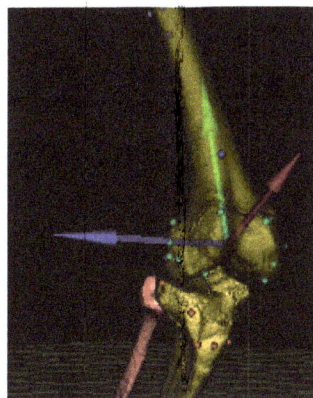

Virtual palpation of skeletal landmarks.

Manual palpation of skeletal landmarks (illustrated here on a patient's shoulder, see left image). The gauntlet on the palpating hand (left) allows to locate the spatial coordinates of the palpated landmarks with a satisfactory accuracy (below 1 cm). Reflective markers are part of the scientific protocol and allow further quantified motion analysis for joint disorders follow-up. *Virtual palpation* of skeletal landmarks located on a 3D bone models (illustrated here on a patient's knee model obtained from medical imaging, see right image). Colored spheres on bones indicate palpated skeletal landmarks. This method combined with quantified manual palpation allows subject-specific visualization of joint behavior during particular motion tasks (e.g., walking, stair climbing, etc.).

The above protocols can be used independently. *Manual palpation* is used in clinical activities for various aims: - identification of painful areas; - positioning of particular pieces of equipment (electromyography electrodes, auscultation, external landmarks used in clinical motion analysis or body surface scanning); or - measurements of morphological parameters (e.g., limb length). *Virtual palpation* alone is useful to quantify individual morphological parameters from medical imaging: - limb length; - limb orientation; - joint angle; or - distance between various skeletal locations.

Combining data from both manual and virtual palpation protocols allows achieving supplementary analysis: - registration protocols aiming at building reference frames for motion representation according reproducible clinical conventions; - to modelize joint kinematics accurately during musculoskeletal analysis; - to align precisely orthopedic tools according to the individual anatomy of a patient; or - to wrap and to scale surface textures to motion data when creating animation characters.

Use of standardized definitions for the above activities allows better result comparison and exchange; this is a key element for patient follow-up, or the elaboration of quality clinical and research databases. Such definitions also allow acceptable repeat ability by individuals with different backgrounds (physiotherapists, medical doctors, nurses, engineers, etc.). If applied strictly, these definitions allow better data exchange and result comparison thanks to standardization of the procedure. Without anatomical landmark standardization, palpation is prone to error and poorly reproducible.

Elastography

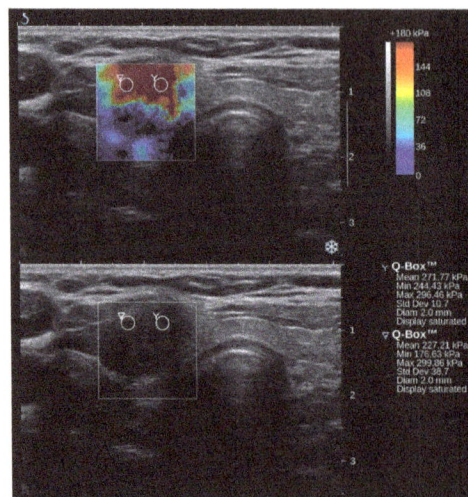

Conventional ultrasonography (lower image) and elastography (supersonic shear imaging; upper image) of papillary thyroid carcinoma, a malignant cancer. The cancer (red) is much stiffer than the healthy tissue.

Nowadays, the medical imaging modality of elastography can also be used to determine the stiffness of tissues. Manual palpation suffers from several important limitations: it is limited to tissues accessible to the physician's hand, it is distorted by any intervening tissue, and it is qualitative but not quantitative. Elastography is able to overcome many these challenges and improve on the benefits of palpation.

Elastography is a relatively new technology, and entered the clinic primarily in the last decade. The most prominent techniques use ultrasound or magnetic resonance imaging (MRI) to make both the stiffness map and an anatomical image for comparison.

Computerized Palpation

While not widespread amongst elastography methods, computerized palpation is of interest here because it essentially uses palpation to measure the stiffness, whereas other techniques will obtain data using other methods. Computerized palpation is also called "Tactile Imaging", "Mechanical imaging" or "Stress imaging", is a medical imaging modality that translates the sense of touch into a digital image. The tactile image is a function of $P(x,y,z)$, where P is the pressure on soft tissue surface under applied deformation and x,y,z are coordinates where pressure P was measured. Tactile imaging closely mimics manual palpation, since the probe of the device with a pressure sensor array mounted on its face acts similar to human fingers during clinical examination, slightly deforming soft tissue by the probe and detecting resulting changes in the pressure pattern.

Palpation under General Anesthesia

Palpation under general anesthesia is sometimes necessary, such as when there is a need to palpate structures deep in the abdominal or pelvic cavity, since it would otherwise cause considerable patient discomfort and subsequent contraction of the abdominal muscles which would make the examination difficult. It is used, for example, in the staging of cervical cancer.

Auscultation

Auscultation (based on the Latin verb *auscultare* "to listen") is listening to the internal sounds of the body, usually using a stethoscope. Auscultation is performed for the purposes of examining the circulatory and respiratory systems (heart and breath sounds), as well as the gastrointestinal system (bowel sounds).

The term was introduced by René-Théophile-Hyacinthe Laënnec. The act of listening to body sounds for diagnostic purposes has its origin further back in history, possibly as early as Ancient Egypt. Laënnec's contributions were refining the procedure, linking sounds with specific pathological changes in the chest, and inventing a suitable instrument (the stethoscope) in the process. Originally, there was a distinction between immediate auscultation (unaided) and mediate auscultation (using an instrument).

Auscultation is a skill that requires substantial clinical experience, a fine stethoscope and good listening skills. Health professionals (doctors, nurses, etc.) listen to three main organs and organ systems during auscultation: the heart, the lungs, and the gastrointestinal system. When auscultating the heart, doctors listen for abnormal sounds, including heart murmurs, gallops, and other extra sounds coinciding with heartbeats. Heart rate is also noted. When listening to lungs, breath sounds such as wheezes, crepitations and crackles are identified. The gastrointestinal system is auscultated to note the presence of bowel sounds.

Electronic stethoscopes can be recording devices, and can provide noise reduction and signal enhancement. This is helpful for purposes of telemedicine (remote diagnosis) and teaching. This opened the field to computer-aided auscultation.

Auscultogram

The sounds of auscultation can be depicted using symbols to produce an auscultogram. It is used in cardiology training.

Immediate auscultation

Immediate auscultation is an antiquated medical term for listening (auscultation) to the internal sounds of the body, directly placing the ear on the body. It is opposed to mediate auscultation, using an instrument (mediate) i.e. a stethoscope.

Mediate Auscultation

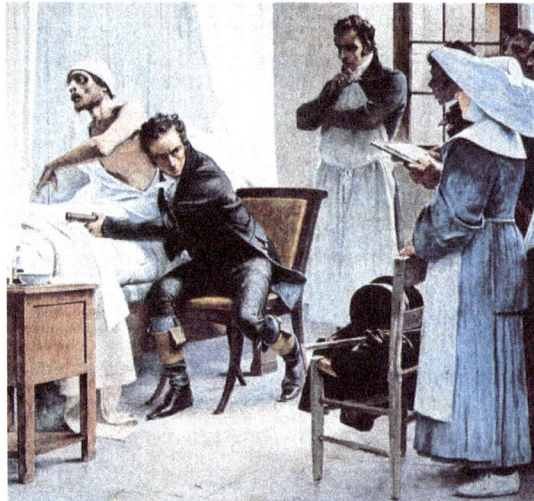

Laennec auscultates a patient before his students.

Mediate auscultation is an antiquated medical term for listening (auscultation) to the internal sounds of the body using an instrument (mediate), usually a stethoscope. It is opposed to immediate auscultation, directly placing the ear on the body.

Doppler Auscultation

It is recently demonstrated that continuous Doppler enables the auscultation of valvular movements and blood flow sounds that are undetected during cardiac examination with a stethoscope in adults. The Doppler auscultation presented a sensitivity of 84% for the detection of aortic regurgitations while classic stethoscope auscultation presented a sensitivity of 58%. Moreover, Doppler auscultation was superior in the detection of impaired ventricular relaxation. Since the physics of

Doppler auscultation and classic auscultation are different, it has been suggested that both methods could complement each other.

Percussion (Medicine)

Percussion is a method of tapping on a surface to determine the underlying structure, and is used in clinical examinations to assess the condition of the thorax or abdomen. It is one of the five methods of clinical examination, together with inspection, palpation, auscultation, and inquiry. It is done with the middle finger of one hand tapping on the middle finger of the other hand using a wrist action. The nonstriking finger (known as the pleximeter) is placed firmly on the body over tissue. When percussing boney areas such as the clavicle the pleximeter can be omitted and the bone is tapped directly such as when percussing an apical cavitary lung lesion typical of TB.

There are two types of percussion: direct, which uses only one or two fingers, and indirect, which uses the middle/flexor finger. There are four types of percussion sounds: resonant, hyper-resonant, stony dull or dull. A dull sound indicates the presence of a solid mass under the surface. A more resonant sound indicates hollow, air-containing structures. As well as producing different notes which can be heard they also produce different sensations in the pleximeter finger.

Percussion was at first used to distinguish between empty and filled barrels of liquor, and Dr. Leopold Auenbrugger is said to be the person who introduced the technique to modern medicine although this method was used by Avicenna about 1000 years before that for medical practice such as using percussion over the stomach to show how full it is and to distinguish between ascites and tympanites.

Of the Thorax

It is used to diagnose pneumothorax, emphysema and other diseases. It can be used to assess the respiratory mobility of the thorax.

Of the Abdomen

It is used to find whether any organ is enlarged and similar (assessing for organomegaly). It is based on the principle of setting tissue and spaces in between at vibration. The sound thus generated is used to determine if the tissue is healthy or pathological.

Based on the auditory and tactile perception, the notes heard can be categorized as:

- Tympanitic, drum-like sounds heard over air filled structures during the abdominal examination.
- Hyperresonant (pneumothorax) said to sound similar to percussion of puffed up cheeks.
- Normal resonance/ Resonant the sound produced by percussing a normal chest.
- Impaired resonance (mass, consolidation) lower than normal percussion sounds.
- Dull (consolidation) similar to percussion of a mass such as a liver.
- Stony dull the sounds produced on percussion from the pleximeter with no contribution from the underlying area.

Percussion may induce pain, this is often also noted as it can indicate underlying pathology.

Nursing Diagnosis

A nursing diagnosis may be part of the nursing process and is a clinical judgment about individual, family, or community experiences/responses to actual or potential health problems/life processes. Nursing diagnoses are developed based on data obtained during the nursing assessment. An actual nursing diagnosis presents a problem response present at time of assessment. Whereas a medical diagnosis identifies a disorder, a nursing diagnosis identifies problems that result from that disorder. The North American Nursing Diagnosis Association (NANDA) is body of professionals that manage an official list of nursing diagnosis.

All nurses must be familiar with the steps of the nursing process in order to gain the most efficiency from their positions.

NANDA International

NANDA-International formerly known as the North American Nursing Diagnosis Association is the primary organization for defining, distribution and integration of standardized nursing diagnoses worldwide. NANDA-I has worked in this area for nearly 40 years to ensure that diagnoses are developed through a peer-reviewed process requiring standardised levels of evidence, definitions, defining characteristics, related factors and/or risk factors that enable nurses to identify potential diagnoses in the course of a nursing assessment. NANDA-I believes that it is critical that nurses are required to utilise standardised languages that provide not just terms (diagnoses) but the embedded knowledge from clinical practice and research that provides diagnostic criteria (definitions, defining characteristics) and the related or etiologic factors upon which nurses intervene. NANDA-I terms are developed and refined for actual (current) health responses and for risk situations, as well as providing diagnoses to support health promotion. Diagnoses are applicable to individuals, families, groups and communities. The taxonomy is published in multiple countries and has been translated into 18 languages; it is in use worldwide.

Nursing diagnoses are a critical part of ensuring that the knowledge and contribution of nursing practice to patient outcomes are found within the electronic health record and can be linked to nurse-sensitive patient outcomes.

Global

The ICNP (International Classification for Nursing Practice) published by the International Council of Nurses has been accepted by the WHO (World Health Organisation) family of classifications. ICNP is a nursing language which can be used by nurses to diagnose.

Structure

The NANDA-I system of nursing diagnosis provides for four categories.

1. Actual diagnosis

    A clinical judgment about human experience/responses to health conditions/life processes that exist in an individual, family, or community. An example of an actual nursing diagnosis is: *Sleep deprivation.*

2. Risk diagnosis

    Describes human responses to health conditions/life processes that may develop in a vulnerable individual/family/community. It is supported by risk factors that contribute to increased vulnerability. An example of a risk diagnosis is: *Risk for shock.*

3. Health promotion diagnosis

    A clinical judgment about a person's, family's or community's motivation and desire to increase wellbeing and actualise human health potential as expressed in the readiness to enhance specific health behaviours, and can be used in any health state. An example of a health promotion diagnosis is: *Readiness for enhanced nutrition.*

4. Syndrome diagnosis

    A clinical judgment describing a specific cluster of nursing diagnoses that occur together, and are best addressed together and through similar interventions. An example of a syndrome diagnosis is: *Relocation stress syndrome.*

Process

1. Assessment

    The first step of the nursing process is assessment. During this phase, the nurse gathers information about a patients psychological, physiological, sociological, and spiritual status. This data can be collected in a variety of ways. Generally, nurses will conduct a patient interview. Physical examinations, referencing a patient's health history, obtaining a patient's family history, and general observation can also be used to gather assessment data. Patient interaction is generally the heaviest during this evaluative stage.

2. Diagnosis

    The diagnosing phase involves a nurse making an educated judgement about a potential or actual health problem with a patient. Multiple diagnoses are sometimes made for a single patient. These assessments not only include a description of the problem or illness (e.g. sleep deprivation) but also whether or not a patient is at risk of developing further problems. These diagnoses are also used to determine a patient's readiness for health improvement and whether or not they may have developed a syndrome. The diagnoses phase is a critical step as it is used to determine the course of treatment.

3. Planning

    Once a patient and nurse agree of the diagnoses, a plan of action can be developed. If multiple diagnoses need to be addressed, the head nurse will prioritise each assessment and devote attention to severe symptoms and high risk patients. Each problem is assigned a clear, measurable goal for the expected beneficial outcome. For this phase, nurses generally refer to the evidence-based Nursing Outcome Classification, which is a set of standardised terms and measurements for tracking patient wellness. The Nursing Interventions Classification may also be used as a resource for planning.

4. Implementation

The implementing phase is where the nurse follows through on the decided plan of action. This plan is specific to each patient and focuses on achievable outcomes. Actions involved in a nursing care plan include monitoring the patient for signs of change or improvement, directly caring for the patient or performing necessary medical tasks, educating and instructing the patient about further health management, and referring or contacting the patient for a follow-up. Implementation can take place over the course of hours, days, weeks, or even months.

5. Evaluation

Once all nursing intervention actions have taken place, the nurse completes an evaluation to determine if the goals for patient wellness have been met. The possible patient outcomes are generally described under three terms: patient;s condition improved, patient's condition stabilised, and patient's condition deteriorated. In the event where the condition of the patient has shown no improvement, or if the wellness goals were not met, the nursing process begins again from the first step.

Examples

The following are nursing diagnoses arising from the nursing literature with varying degrees of authentication by ICNP or NANDA-I standards.

- Anxiety

- Constipation

- Pain

Nursing Care Plan

A nursing care plan provides direction on the type of nursing care the individual/family/community may need . The main focus of a nursing care plan is to facilitate standardised, evidence-based and holistic care. Nursing care plans have been used for quite a number of years for human purposes and are now also getting used in the veterinary profession. The Care Plan includes the following components; assessment, diagnosis, expected outcomes, interventions, rationale and evaluation. According to Ballantyne care plans are a critical aspect of nursing and they are meant to allow standardised, evidence-based holistic care. It is important to draw attention to the difference between 'care plan' and 'care planning'. Care planning is related to identifying problems and coming up with solutions to reduce or remove the problems. The care plan is essentially the documentation of this process. It includes within it a set of actions the nurse will apply to resolve/support nursing diagnoses identified by nursing assessment. Care plans make it possible for interventions to be recorded and their effectiveness assessed. Nursing care plans provide continuity of care, safety, quality care and compliance. Nursing care plans promotes documentation and is used for reimbursement purposes such as Medicare and Medicaid.

Objective

1. To promote evidence-based care

2. To promote holistic care which means the whole person is considered including physical, psychological, social and spiritual in relation to management and prevention of the disease.

3. To support methods such as care pathways and care bundles. Care pathways involve a team effort in order to come to a consensus with regards to standards of care and expected outcomes while care bundles are related to best practice with regards to care given for a specific disease.

4. To record care.

5. To measure care.

Characteristics

1. Its' focus is holistic, and is based on the clinical judgment of the nurse, using assessment data collected from a nursing framework.

2. It is based upon identifiable nursing diagnoses (actual, risk or health promotion) - clinical judgments about individual, family, or community experiences/responses to actual or potential health problems/life processes.

3. It focuses on client-specific nursing outcomes that are realistic for the care recipient.

4. It includes nursing interventions which are focused on the etiologic or risk factors of the identified nursing diagnoses.

5. It is a product of a deliberate systematic process.

Components of a Care Plan

A care plan includes the following components;

1. Client assessment, medical results and diagnostic reports. This is the first step in order to be able to create a care plan. In particular client assessment is related to the following areas and abilities: physical, emotional, sexual, psychosocial, cultural, spiritual/ transpersonal, cognitive, functional, age related, economic and environmental. Information is this area can be subjective and objective.

2. Expected patient outcomes are outlined. These may be long and short term.

3. Nursing interventions are documented in the Care Plan.

4. Rationale for interventions in order to be evidence based care.

5. Evaluation. This documents the outcome of nursing interventions.

Computerised Nursing Care Plans

A computerised nursing care plan is a digital way of writing the care plan, compared to handwritten. Computerised nursing care plans are an essential element of the nursing process. Computerised nursing care plans have increased documentation of signs and symptoms, associated factors and nursing interventions. Using electronic devices when creating nursing care plans are a more accurate, accessible, easier completed and easier edited, in comparison with handwritten and pre-printed care plans.

References

- Katz, S; Stroud M (1963). "Functional assessment in geriatrics: a review of progress and direction". Journal of the American Geriatrics Society. 37: 267–271

- Chinn, Peggy; Kramer, Maeona (November 30, 2010). Integrated Theory & Knowledge Development in Nursing (8 ed.). St. Louis: Mosby. ISBN 0323077188

- Natt, B; Szerlip, HM (2014), "The lost art of the history and physical", Am J Med Sci, 348 (5): 423–425, doi:10.1097/MAJ.0000000000000326, PMID 25247755

- Alligood, Martha Raile, ed. (2014-01-01). Nursing theory: utilization & application (5 ed.). St. Louis, Missouri: Elsevier Mosby. ISBN 9780323091893

- Krogsbøll, Lasse T; Jørgensen, Karsten Juhl (2012). "General health checks in adults for reducing morbidity and mortality from disease". Cochrane: 1. doi:10.1002/14651858.CD009009.pub2

- Barnum, Barbara (1998). Nursing Theory: Analysis, Application, Evaluation. Lippincott Williams & Wilkins. ISBN 978-0-7817-1104-3

- Mahoney, F; Barthel D (1965). "Functional evaluation: the Barthel index". Maryland State Medical Journal. 14: 61–65. PMID 14258950

- George, Julia B. (2011). Nursing Theories: The Base for Professional Nursing Practice, 6th Ed. Upper Saddle River, NJ: Pearson. p. 213. ISBN 978-0-13-513583-9

- "Diagnostic errors are leading cause of successful malpractice claims". The Washington Post. 2012-04-30. Retrieved 2016-10-31

- Verghese A, Horwitz RI (2009). "In praise of the physical examination" (PDF). BMJ. 339: b5448. doi:10.1136/bmj.b5448. PMID 20015910

- Office, Publications. "SNOMED CT - Systematized Nomenclature of Medicine". sydney.edu.au. Retrieved 17 January 2017

- Verghese A, Brady E, Kapur CC, Horwitz RI (October 2011). "The bedside evaluation: ritual and reason". Ann. Intern. Med. 155 (8): 550–3. doi:10.7326/0003-4819-155-8-201110180-00013. PMID 22007047

- Siviter, B. (2008) Student Nurse Handbook: a survivial guide 2nd edition, Edinburgh: Balliere Tindall for Elsevier ISBN 978-0-7020-2946-2

- "Comprehensive Nursing Assessment" (PDF). Department of Mental Health and Hygiene. Maryland.gov. 6 June 2012. Retrieved 9 November 2016

- Roper N., Logan W.W. & Tierney A.J. (2000). The Roper-Logan-Tierney Model of Nursing: Based on Activities of Living. Edinburgh: Elsevier Health Sciences. ISBN 0-443-06373-7

3

Types of Nursing Specialties

The different types of nursing are surgical nursing, flight nurse, obstetrical nursing, nurse anesthetist, peranesthesia nursing and certified nurse midwife. Surgical nurse provides care to the patient during the surgery and after it as well. Obstetrical nurses are nurses who work with women who are pregnant or are trying to conceive. The major types of nursing specialties are dealt with great details in the chapter.

Surgical Nursing

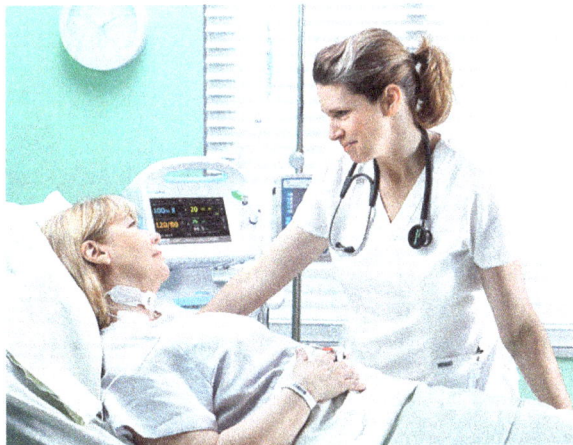

Image sourced from the medGadget. This is an example of post operative care.

A surgical nurse, also referred to as a theatre nurse or scrub nurse, specializes in preoperative care, providing care to patients before, during and after surgery. To become a theatre nurse, Registered Nurses or Enrolled Nurses must complete extra training. There are different speciality areas that theatre nurses can focus in depending on which areas they are interested in.

There are many different phases during surgery where the theatre nurse is needed to support and assist the patient, surgeons, surgical technicians, nurse anaesthetists and nurse practitioners. Pre-operative, the nurse must help to prepare the patient and operating room for the surgery. During the surgery, they assist the anaesthetist and surgeons when they are needed. The last phase is post-operative, enduring that the patients are provided with suitable care and treatments.

People who want to become surgical nurses attend nursing school and specialize in surgical nursing. They are often required to pass examinations administered by the government or by nursing certification boards before being allowed to work as nurses, and they may also be expected to attend periodic continuing education classes so that they keep up with developments in the nursing field.

Surgical patients (those who have undergone a minor or major surgical procedure) are nursed on different wards to medical patients in the UK and Australia. Nursing practice on surgical wards differs from that of medical wards.

Surgical nurses may practice in different types of surgery:

- General surgery (e.g. appendectomy, gallbladder removal)
- Vascular surgery (e.g. varicose vein surgery, aortic aneurysm repair)
- Colo-rectal surgery (e.g. stoma formation)
- Surgical Oncology (e.g. breast surgery, tumour resections)
- Orthopaedic surgery (e.g. knee or hip replacements, fracture repair)
- Urological surgery (e.g. prostate surgery)
- Day surgery (or ambulatory surgery, where a patient is discharged within 24 hours)

Surgical nurses are responsible for approximately six patients, depending on the nature of the surgical ward. Intensive Care and High-Dependency units usually have one to two nurses per patient.

Duties

Theatre nurses are part of the perioperative surgical team, they work alongside surgeons, surgical technician, nurse anaesthetists and nurse practitioners.

In surgery there are 3 main phases: preoperative, intraoperative and postoperative. These phases collectively are known as the perioperative period. Perioperative nursing is the way by which nursing care is provided. Each phase is related to specific activities carried out and skills needed for different stages of nursing.

Preoperative Phase

This stage is undertaken when the patient decides to have surgery. Preoperative phase, which includes discussing to the patients about all the benefits of the procedure but also the dangers that could occur. By giving this information to the patients prior their operation, it's a good chance for the patient to discuss any concerns they may have. Also the theatre nurses must making sure that the patients are in good health, before going ahead with the surgery. While it is very important to prepare a patient physically it is also important to mentally prepare a patient prior to surgery. A surgical nurse will help prepare the patient using various methods often including family members depending on the situation. The patient will normally express any concerns about the surgery to the nurse, this information will be passed on to other hospital staff including the surgeon, the appropriate actions will be taken dependant on the situation.

Intraoperative Phase

This stage begins when the ward nurse, who has prepared the patient for surgery, delivers the patient and their notes to the theatre and/or anaesthetic nurse. Many checks are undertaken in this stage to ensure a safe environment for the patient and the theatre staff. The theatre nurse carries out activities to maintain a sterile environment and to ensure the surgical equipment is working well. The nurse also organises all surgical instruments and ensures all supplies needed during the surgery are available.

Postoperative Phase

This phase begins when the theatre/anaesthetic nurse delivers the patients notes to the nurses and staff in the Post-Anaesthetic Care Unit (PACU). This can also be known as the recovery room. Here the nurse's immediate attention is on checking the patient's airway and breathing. In this phase nurses also attend to pain relief and any other complications following surgery. These nurses, often in day surgery cases, attend to provide patients and their caregivers with support and instructions and requirements needed for home care.

The first twenty-four hours post surgery are critical, there are many procedures that should take place in order to monitor the patient. Observations of the patient need to be taken and recorded every fifteen minutes. General observations are inclusive of, heart rate, blood pressure, temperature, respiratory rate and oxygen saturation. Further tasks taken out by a surgical nurse post operation include; urine output, assessment of wound sites, replacing intravenous requirements and reporting any abnormalities. It is also a task of the nurse to collect information about the social patient's history or issues, mobility restrictions, nutrition and education requirements prior to discharge from hospital. When these tasks are taken out it is proven to improve recovery.

Credentials

To become a surgical nurse,CCTC one must have undertaken appropriate training, and be registered with the state nursing board (Nursing and Midwifery Council, UK; An Bord Altranais, Rep. of Ireland). In Australia, both Registered Nurses and Enrolled Nurses work in surgical wards. Registered nursing received their training over a longer period of time, as they receive a University degree. To become a registered nurse you must complete a bachelor's degree of nursing which takes up to 3 years. Enrolled Nurses complete a Diploma of Nursing which is a full-time course over 12 –16 months at Technical and Further Education (TAFE).

In Australia, the education standards are nationwide, requiring an undergraduate nursing degree and graduate diploma in perioperative nursing. The undergraduate degree has a full-time study duration of three years at the University of Notre Dame. The post graduate diploma in preoperative nursing has some prerequisites including; undergraduate nursing degree, be a full-time employee of the Fremantle Health Service, hold a current licence to practice as a level one registered nurse and have at least one year of postgraduate experience. With these qualifications it is possible to become a surgical nurse in Australia.

The Graduate Diploma in Perioperative Nursing is available 1 year full-time or equivalent part-time and is developed to qualify the registered nurse to enhance knowledge and combine skills to work as a specialist within the perioperative field.

Types of Surgical Nurse

In the theatre room there are two main types of nurses, a scrub nurse and a circulation nurse. The scrub nurses job is to make sure they are familiar and well educated with every piece of operational equipment. As on request they are required to provide the surgeons with the equipment needed. The scrub nurse is also responsible for making sure all operating equipment is accounted for before and after the operation.

The scrub nurse is responsible for many important technical duties. These can include ensuring they have correctly prepared the surgical instruments and trolleys and ensuring that all operating supplies have been sterilised. Other skills significantly important for the scrub nurse role include non-technical skills. These can include cognitive skills such as formulating appropriate decisions. Another non-technical skill required is being able to work well within a team, for example, the ability to communicate well with the surgical team during a procedure.

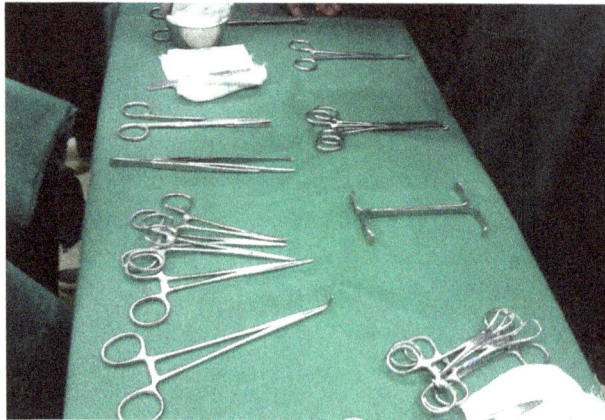
Surgical instruments on a trolley in preparation for surgery

A circulation nurse have many similar responsible, although they are to insure that the operating room is clear and non-contaminated by previous surgeries or other infections. They are also there to collected, open, clear and sterilise packets containing surgical equipment.

Surgical Nurse Interaction with Patients

It is important for surgical nurses to have a thorough understanding of their roles and interactions with patients and their immediate families within a surgical care environment. One vital role for a surgical nurse is to provide support and confidence to their patient while they are in hospital. Nurses are also required to possess good communication skills and maintain a professional relationship with their patient. It is important for the nurse to build a trusting relationship with their patient but this can prove difficult within the short time available. Due to the fast-paced surgical surroundings, there is little time for surgical nurses to provide information and reassurance before and after surgery. Many patients feel vulnerable and anxious prior to their surgical procedure and it is important for the surgical nurse to recognise their patient's need for psychological support. It is therefore important for the surgical nurse to understand their role in relation to the patient. By understanding the emotional needs of their patients, surgical nurses' perspectives and conduct towards their patient will influence the patient's experience.

Preoperative Teaching

Preoperative teaching if delivered competently is an important aspect of patient care. Positive effects of preoperative teaching include a reduction in patients' anxiety levels, healing time, complications post- surgery, pain relief usage and an increase in satisfied and co-operative patient's in regard to their procedure and treatment. Preoperative teaching is essential to a patient's understanding of the surgical procedure and to help them prepare for postoperative healing.

Preoperative teaching is usually undertaken before the day of surgery. This can be delivered by verbal and/or written instructions. Patients may also have an appointment scheduled with the perioperative nurse to talk over any concerns regarding the procedure. Teaching is further discussed on the day of surgery and also before the patient is discharged to leave the hospital.

Potential Careers

Nurses who work in the operating theatre become specialists in the field or a specific sub speciality. Once you find a specialist field or specific sub speciality you enjoy working in, the nurse will commence as a junior nurse. After gaining a large amount of knowledge and skills set with experience, if the nurse chooses to become more of an expert in this field. The theatre nurse may do a postgraduate certificate or diploma to become a Clinical Nurse for that speciality. The salary for a surgical nurse in Australia can range from $47,721 to $80,160 with an average of $57,103 this data was recorded in March 2016.

Professional Associations - Perioperative Nursing Associations

The role of professional associations is to protect, increase and promote common interests of their members. They provide opportunities such as networking, clinical education and research grants. Each Australian State has their own group which form a subdivision of ACORN (Australian College of Perioperative Nurses). Western Australia's group is the Operating Nurses Association of Western Australia (ORNA). Both ACORN and ORNA have a website which provides information about their organisation.

Flight Nurse

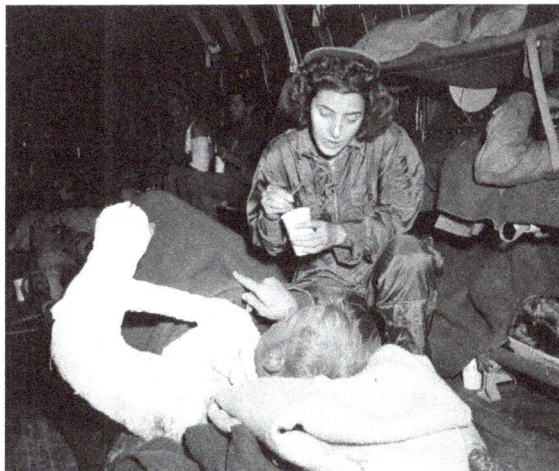

The first United States Navy Flight Nurse, Jane Kendeigh

A Flight Nurse is a registered nurse who specialises in the field of providing comprehensive pre-hospital, emergency critical care and hospital care to a vast scope of patients. The care of these patients is generally during aeromedical evacuation or rescue operations aboard helicopters, propeller aircraft or jet aircraft. On-board a rescue aircraft you would find a flight nurse accompanied by flight medics and respiratory practitioners, as well as the option of a flight physician for comprehensive emergency and critical transport teams. The inclusion of a flight physician is more commonly seen in pediatric and neonatal transport teams.

Roles and Duties

A Flight Nurse is required to complete a copious amount of duties each and every call out. Listed below is a comprehensive list of these duties and responsibilities:

- Flight Nurses perform as a member of an aeromedical evacuation team on helicopters and propeller or jet aircraft

- Responsible for planning and preparing for aeromedical evacuation missions

- Expedite mission and initiate emergency treatment in absence of Flight Physician

- Provide in-flight management and nursing care for patients

- Evaluate individual patient in-flight needs

- Liaison between medical and operational aircrews and support personnel to promote patient comfort

- Responsible for maintaining patient care, comfort and safety

- Care for patients with both medical and traumatic issues

- Request appropriate medications, supplies and equipment to provide care to patient

- Must have training in mechanical ventilation, hemodynamic support, vasoactive medications and intensive care skills

- Specialised clinical skills in union with knowledge, theory, education and expertise in hospital and pre-hospital environments are required

- Perform advanced medical procedures without supervision of a doctor such as intubation, ventilator management, chest tube insertion, intra-osseous line placement, central line placement, intra-aortic balloon pump management, management of pacing devices, titration of vasoactive medications, pain management, administration of anaesthetic medications for intubation, and in some cases, emotional and family care

Education

National Requirements for most Flight Nurse Programs Include

- License as a registered nurse- attainable through most Universities or Education Institutions

- 2–3 years of critical care experience and/or Mobile Intensive Care Unit (MICU) experience.

- Advanced Cardiac Life Support certificate (ACLS)

- Pediatric Advanced Life Support Certificate (PALS)

Additional requirements may include:

- Neonatal Resuscitation Program (NRP)

- Nationally recognised trauma program such as Pre Hospital Trauma Life (PHTLS)

- Support (PHTLS), Basic Trauma Life Support (BTLS), Trauma Nurse Core Course (TNCC), or Transport Nurse Advanced Trauma Course (TNATC)

- Certifications such as Critical Care certification (CCRN), Certified Emergency Nurse (CEN), or Certified Flight Registered Nurse (CFRN)

Helpful, but may not be required:

- EMT or EMT-P (Paramedic) certification with field experience (some states require flight nurses to be certified as EMT's or EMT-P's)

Credentialing

- Certified Emergency Nurse (CEN)

- Certified Flight Registered Nurse (CFRN)

- Critical Care Registered Nurse (CCRN)

Types of Flight Nurses

Civilian Flight Nurse

- Works for hospitals, federal, state and local governments, private medical evacuation firms, fire departments and other agencies.

Military Flight Nurse

- Army Air Force Evacuation Service

- Member of aeromedical evacuation crew

- Senior medical member of aeromedical evacuation team on Continental United States (CONUS)

- Works in intra-theatre and inter-theatre flights to provide in-flight management and nursing care

- Plan/Prepare aeromedical evacuation missions and prepare patient care facilitation plan

Australian Flight Nursing

Australia has an estimated 20% of land recognised as desert with a rather small population density. Providing health care to these remote, rural towns can prove to be quite laborious. Australia provides a number of organisations that flight nurses are under employment of.

Extra Reading

Several books and weblink have been published to give an insight into Flight Nursing, some of these include:

- Operation Flight Nurse: Real-Life Medical Emergencies (Kaniecki, 2013)

- Trauma Junkie: Memoirs of an Emergency Flight Nurse (Hudson, 2010)

- RAF Medical Services

- Air Medical Services

- Royal Flying Doctor Service of Australia

Perioperative Nursing

Perioperative nursing is a nursing specialty that works with patients who are having operative or other invasive procedures. Perioperative nurses work closely with surgeons, anaesthesiologists, nurse anaesthetists, surgical technologists, and nurse practitioners. They perform preoperative, intraoperative, and postoperative care primarily in the operating theatre.

Perioperative Nursing Roles

Perioperative nurses in Australia may perform several roles, including circulating, instrument (or scrub) nurse, preoperative (or patient reception) nurse, Post Anaesthetic Care Unit or recovery nurse, registered nurse first assistant (RNFA), and patient educator

Circulating Nurse

The circulating nurse is a perioperative nurse who assists in managing the nursing care of a patient during surgery. The circulating nurse observes for breaches in surgical asepsis and coordinates the needs of the surgical team. The circulating nurse is not scrubbed in the case, but rather manages the care and environment during surgery

Instrument Nurse

An instrument (scrub) nurse is a perioperative nurse who works directly with the surgeon within the sterile field. The instrument nurse manages the sterile equipment, anticipates the surgeon's needs, and passes instruments and other items required during the procedure. Other duties include surgical site skin preparation, sterile draping, suctioning, irrigation, and retraction. The title comes from the requirement to scrub their hands and arms with special disinfecting solutions.

RN First Assistant

An RNFA is the surgeon's assistant and is extremely qualified in providing extended perioperative nursing care. The role also includes preoperative, intraoperative, and postoperative care of the patient.

Perianaesthesia Nursing

The perianaesthesia nurse (recovery nurse) provides intensive nursing care to patients after they wake from anaesthesia. This nurse cares for and monitors patients to make sure they are not nauseous or disoriented.

Obstetrical Nursing

Obstetrical nursing, also called perinatal nursing, is a nursing specialty that works with patients who are attempting to become pregnant, are currently pregnant, or have recently delivered. Obstetrical nurses help provide prenatal care and testing, care of patients experiencing pregnancy complications, care during labor and delivery, and care of patients following delivery. Obstetrical nurses work closely with obstetricians, midwives, and nurse practitioners. They also provide supervision of patient care technicians and surgical technologists.

Obstetrical nurses perform postoperative care on a surgical unit, stress test evaluations, cardiac monitoring, vascular monitoring, and health assessments. Obstetrical nurses are required to possess specialized skills such as electronic fetal monitoring, nonstress tests, neonatal resuscitation, and medication administration by continuous intravenous drip.

Obstetrical nurses work in many different environments such as medical offices, prenatal clinics, labor & delivery units, antepartum units, postpartum units, operating theatres, and clinical research.

In the U.S. and Canada, the professional nursing organization for obstetrical nurses is the Association of Women's Health, Obstetric and Neonatal Nursing (AWHONN).

Certification for Obstetrical Nurses

The National Certification Corporation (NCC) offers certifications for obstetrical nurses. These include RNC-OB (Inpatient Obstetrics), a certification that allows graduate nurses who have completed a bachelor's degree in the US or Canada, who want to expand into obstetrics. It is an online exam that costs around $325, and by the end of it they will gain themselves RNC-OB certificates. RNC-MNN (Maternal Newborn Nursing) is another online exam that is for certified registered nurses, who have completed their bachelor's degrees in Nursing and have gained experienced in the area of newborn nursing, and are wanting to gain a certification/qualification in the area. The test costs around $325 and they have a 90-day window to complete the actual exam and C-EFM (Electronic Fetal Monitoring). This certification like the other two is an online citification exam, for US and Canadian graduate nursing students. To do the online certification they are required to be either a licensed registered nurse, nurse practitioner, nurse midwife, physician, physician assistant, or paramedic, according to the US and Canada requirements.

Australian Certification and Requirements

Bachelor's degrees in either nursing and/or midwifery are required to become an obstetrical or perinatal nurse in Australia. In Australia alone there are 32 different universities that offer nursing as an undergraduate degree, such as Australian Catholic university, Charles Darwin University and the University of Notre Dame in Australia. Once completing their degree, they are required to complete their master's degree in nursing. Bachelor's degrees and jobs as licensed nurses/midwives are required in order to be accepted for the master's degree. There are 24 different universities in Australia that offer a master's degree in nursing, including Edith Cowan University, Monash University, James Cook University and University of Canberra.

Oncology Nursing

An oncology nurse is a specialized nurse who cares for cancer patients.

Certification in the United States

The Oncology Nursing Certification Corporation (ONCC) offers several different options for board certification in oncological nursing. Certification is a voluntary process and ensures that a nurse has proper qualifications and knowledge of a specialty area and has kept up-to-date in his or her education.

The ONCC offers eight options for certification:

- *Basic:*
    - o OCN: Oncology Certified Nurse
    - o CPON: Certified Pediatric Oncology Nurse
    - o CPHON: Certified Pediatric Hematology Oncology Nurse
- *Specialty:*
    - o BMTCN: Blood and Marrow Transplant Certified Nurse
    - o CBCN: Certified Breast Care Nurse
- *Advanced:*
    - o AOCN: Advanced Oncology Certified Nurse

- o   AOCNP: Advanced Oncology Certified Nurse Practitioner

- o   AOCNS: Advanced Oncology Certified Clinical Nurse Specialist

Certification is granted for four years, after which it must be renewed by taking a recertification test or by earning a certain number of continuing education credits.

To become certified, nurses must have an RN license, meet specific eligibility criteria for nursing experience and specialty practice, and must pass a multiple-choice test.

For the advanced AOCNP and AOCNS certifications, a nurse must have a master's degree or higher in nursing and a minimum of 500 hours of supervised clinical practice of oncology nursing. The AOCNP certification also requires successful completion of an accredited nurse practitioner program.

Oncology Nursing in Morocco

Demand

The demand for oncology nurses is enormous in Morocco. Statistics of the Moroccan Ministry of Health indicate that the death toll of malignant neoplasms mounts to 17 thousands a year. The number of patients with cancer is believed to be three-times the number of annual deaths. A recent study of the European Institute of Health Sciences (Institut Européen des Sciences de la Santé) projected that the need for oncology nurses in 2025 is estimated at 5 thousand nurses. Yet, the number of qualified oncology nurses in the country is equal to nil. The reason is obviously the absence of a formal educational program in oncology nursing.

Oncology Nursing Training in Morocco

Currently there currently exists only one educational program in oncology nursing that is being offered by the European Institute of Health Sciences. It has been approved by the Ministry of Higher Education as well as the Ministry of Health in 2014. The duration of this Bachelor of Science program in Oncology Nursing is 3 years and encompasses a total of 6 thousands hours, equivalent to 120 semester credits in the US educational system and 180 ECTS in the European system. The program attracts a large number of students from African countries.

Certification Requirements in Morocco

In Morocco, there exists no system for certification of oncology nurses. However, graduates of the oncology nursing program of the European Institute of Health Sciences can set for certification exams abroad, particularly in European countries.

Telenursing

Telenursing refers to the use of telecommunications and information technology in the provision of nursing services whenever a large physical distance exists between patient and nurse, or between any number of nurses. As a field, it is part of telehealth, and has many points of contacts with other medical and non-medical applications, such as telediagnosis, teleconsultation, telemonitoring, Telemedicine etc.

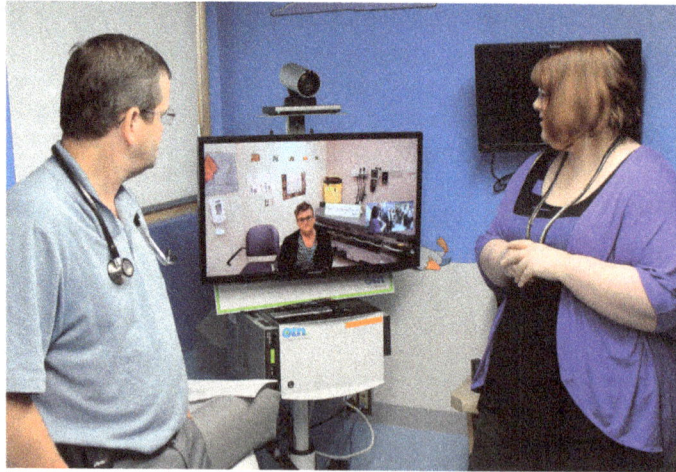

New telecommunication equipment for nurses and doctors at Health Sciences North/Horizon Santé-Nord (HSN) in Ontario, Canada

Telenursing is achieving a large rate of growth in many countries, due to several factors: the preoccupation in driving down the costs of health care, an increase in the number of aging and chronically ill population, and the increase in coverage of health care to distant, rural, small or sparsely populated regions. Among its many benefits, telenursing may help solve increasing shortages of nurses; to reduce distances and save travel time, and to keep patients out of hospital. A greater degree of job satisfaction has been registered among telenurses.

Applications

Home Care

One of the most distinctive telenursing applications is home care. For example, patients who are immobilized, or live in remote or difficult to reach places, citizens who have chronic ailments, such as chronic obstructive pulmonary disease, diabetes, congestive heart disease, or debilitating diseases, such as neural degenerative diseases (Parkinson's disease, Alzheimer's disease or ALS), may stay at home and be "visited" and assisted regularly by a nurse via videoconferencing, internet or videophone. Other applications of home care are the care of patients in immediate post-surgical situations, the care of wounds, ostomies or disabled individuals. In normal home health care, one nurse is able to visit up to 5-7 patients per day. Using telenursing, one nurse can "visit" 12-16 patients in the same amount of time.

Case Management

A common application of telenursing is also used by call centers operated by managed care organizations, which are staffed by registered nurses who act as case managers or perform patient triage, information and counseling as a means of regulating patient access and flow and decrease the use of emergency rooms. McKesson is a leading telephone health service provider in the United States of America, as well as in Australasia.

Telephone Triage

Telephone triage refers to symptom or clinically-based calls. Clinicians perform symptom assessment by asking detailed questions about the patient's illness or injury. The clinician's task is to estimate and/or rule out urgent symptoms. They may use pattern recognition and other problem-solving process as well. Clinicians may utilize guidelines, in paper or electronic format, to determine how urgent the symptoms are. Telephone triage requires clinicians to determine if the symptoms are life-threatening, emergency, urgent, acute or non-acute. It may involve educating and advising clients, and making safe, effective, and appropriate dispositions—all by telephone. Telephone triage takes place in settings as diverse as emergency rooms, ambulance services, large call centers, physician offices, clinics, student health centers and hospices.

Countries using Telephone Triage

An International Telenursing survey was completed in 2005, reporting that the 719 responding full time and part time Registered Nurses and Advanced Practice Nurses worked as a telenurse in 36 countries around the world. 68% of these Telenurses where reported to be working in the United States of America, whereas .6% where to be working in Finland. Some of these 36 counties include;

- Australia

- Canada

- Norway

- United Kingdom

- New Zealand

- Iran

- Sweden

- Netherlands

In Australia

In Australia, telephone triages are conducted in Western Australia, Australian Capital Territory, Northern Territory, Victoria and Queensland. The first telenursing triage was conducted in Western Australia in 1999, where Triage nurses would estimate patient complexity and refer them to Fremantle Hospital. Due to the remoteness of the Australian landscape it is vital that residents living in rural areas have access to clinical support and care. Telenursing allows nurses to overcome the barriers of distance and gives them the opportunity assist those who are unable to access health care clinics or services due to either the late hour or the distance.

Legal, Ethical and Regulatory Issues

Telenursing is fraught with legal, ethical and regulatory issues, as it happens with telehealth as a whole. In many countries, interstate and intercountry practice of telenursing is forbidden (the attending nurse must have a license both in their state/country of residence and in the state/country where the patient receiving telecare is located). The Nurse Licensure Compact helps resolve some of these jurisdiction issues. Legal issues such as accountability and malpractice, etc. are also still largely unsolved and difficult to address. Ethical issues include maintaining autonomy, maintaining a patients integrity as well as preventing harm to a patient.

In addition, there are many considerations related to patient confidentiality and safety of clinical data.

Nurse Anesthetist

A nurse anesthetist is a nurse who specializes in the administration of anesthesia. In the United States, a certified registered nurse anesthetist (CRNA) is an advanced practice registered nurse (APRN) who has acquired graduate-level education and board certification in anesthesia. The American Association of Nurse Anesthetists' (AANA) is the national association that represents more than 90% of the 50,000 nurse anesthetists in the United States. Certification is governed by the National Board of Certification and Recertification for Nurse Anesthetists (NBCRNA). Education is governed by the Council on Accreditation (COA) of Nurse Anesthesia Educational Programs. In order to get into this graduate program, one must obtain a BSN degree in nursing, as well as complete their boards and get a license. The average GPA of students who are accepted into CRNA schools ranges from 3.3 – 3.7. The next step is to have a minimum of one year of acute care experience, for example the ICU.

Worldwide, in the UK and former commonwealth countries, the term anesthetist is used for physicians only. It is the British version for a US anesthesiologist.

In the United States

Nurse anesthetists have been providing anesthesia care in the United States for more than 150 years. According to the American Association of Nurse Anesthetists, nurse anesthetists are the oldest nurse specialty group in the United States. Additionally, in testament to the profession's roots, today's nurse anesthetists remain the primary anesthesia providers to U.S. service men and women at home and abroad.

Among the first American nurses to provide anesthesia was Catherine S. Lawrence. Along with other nurses, Lawrence administered anesthesia during the American Civil War (1861–1865). The first "official" nurse anesthetist is recognized as Sister Mary Bernard, a Catholic nun who practiced in 1877 at St. Vincent's Hospital in Erie, Pennsylvania. There is evidence that up to 50 or more other Catholic sisters were called to practice anesthesia in various midwest Catholic and Protestant hospitals throughout the last two decades of the 19th century. The first school of nurse anesthesia was formed in 1909 at St. Vincent Hospital, Portland, Oregon. Established by Agnes McGee, the course was seven months long, and included courses on anatomy and physiology, pharmacology, and administration of common anesthetic agents. Within the next decade, approximately 19 schools opened. All consisted of post-graduate anesthesia training for nurses and were about six months in length. These included programs at Mayo Clinic, Johns

Hopkins Hospital, Barnes Hospital, New York Post-Graduate Hospital, Charity Hospital in New Orleans, Grace Hospital in Detroit, among others. Early anesthesia training programs provided education for all levels of health providers. For example, in 1915, chief nurse anesthetist Agatha Hodgins established the Lakeside Hospital School of Anesthesia in Cleveland, Ohio. This program was open to nurses, physicians, and dentists. The training was six months and the tuition was $50. A diploma was awarded on completion. In its first year, it graduated six physicians, two dentists, and 11 nurses. Later, in 1918, it established a system of clinical affiliations with other Cleveland hospitals. Some nurse anesthetists were appointed to medical school faculties to train the medical students in anesthesia. For example, Agnes McGee also taught third year medical school students at the Oregon Health Science Center. Furthermore, nurse anesthetist Alice Hunt was appointed instructor in anesthesia with university rank at the Yale University School of Medicine in 1922. She held this position for 26 years. In addition, she authored the 1949 book *Anesthesia, Principles and Practice*. This is most likely the first nurse anesthesia textbook.

Early nurse anesthetists were involved in publications. For example, in 1906, nurse anesthetist Alice Magaw (1860–1928) published a report on the use of ether anesthesia by drop method 14,000 times without a fatality *(Surg., Gynec. & Obst. 3:795, 1906)*. Beginning in 1899, Magaw authored several publications with some published and many ignored because of her status as a non-physician. Ms. Magaw was the anesthetist at St. Mary's Hospital in Rochester for the famous brothers, Dr. William James Mayo and Dr. Charles Horace Mayo. This became the Mayo Clinic in Rochester, Minnesota. Ms. Magaw set up a showcase for surgery and anesthesia that has attracted many students and visitors.

Education Pathway

Nurse Anesthesia is a graduate-prepared profession. In the United States of America, nurse anesthetists must be licensed registered nurse and complete a master's degree in anesthesia and/or nursing with a post-masters certification in anesthesia. In addition, candidates are required to have a minimum of one year of full-time nursing experience in a medical or surgical intensive care unit. Following this experience, applicants apply to a Council on Accreditation of Nurse Anesthesia Educational Programs (COA) accredited program of nurse anesthesia. Education is offered on a master's degree or doctoral degree (in Nurse Anesthesia Practice). Program length is typically 28 months in duration, but can vary from 24 to 36 months. The didactic curricula of nurse-anesthesia programs are governed by the COA standards and provide students the scientific, clinical, and professional foundation upon which to build a sound and safe clinical practice. Accredited programs afford and ensure supervised experiences for students during which time they are able to learn anesthesia techniques, test theory, and apply knowledge to clinical problems. Students gain experience with patients of all ages who require medical, surgical, obstetrical, dental, and pediatric interventions. In addition, many require study in methods of scientific inquiry and statistics, as well as active participation in student-generated and faculty-sponsored research. Among the oldest schools in the U.S., Ravenswood Hospital in Chicago, opened in 1925 by Mae Cameron, which in 2001 became the NorthShore University HealthSystem School of Nurse Anesthesia, was the first school to be accredited by the Council on Accreditation of Nurse Anesthesia Educational Programs in 1952.

History of Education

CRNAs in the United States receive Master's or Doctoral degrees in nurse anesthesia. The Council on Accreditation develops requirements for degree programs. In 1981, the Council on Accreditation developed guidelines for master's degrees. In 1982, it was the official position of the AANA board of directors that registered nurses applying for a school of anesthesia shall be, at minimum, baccalaureate prepared and then complete a master's level anesthesia program. At that time, many programs started phasing in advanced degree requirements. As early as 1978, the Kaiser Permanente California State University program had evolved to a master's level program. All programs were required to transition to a master's degree beginning in 1990 and complete the process by 1998. Currently, the American Association of Colleges of Nursing has endorsed a position statement that will move the current entry level of training and education of nurse anesthetists in the United States to the Doctor of Nursing Practice (DNP) or Doctor of Nurse Anesthesia Practice (DNAP). This move will affect all advance practice nurses, with a mandatory implementation by the year 2015. In August 2007, the AANA announced its support of this advanced clinical degree as an entry level for practice of all nurse anesthetists with a target compliance date of 2025. In accordance with traditional grandfathering rules, all those in current practice will not be affected. Several nurse anesthesia programs have already transitioned to the DNP or DNAP entry level format. Because all programs will be converting to a doctorate level education, the length of the programs will continue to expand. Nurse anesthetists have always embraced the responsibility of helping meet America's growing healthcare needs. As healthcare technologies continue to advance and the knowledge base of the human body continues to expand, the 2025 requirement of a doctoral level education for entry into nurse anesthesia practice will ensure that patients have continued access to the highest quality anesthesia care that is possible.

Certification

The certification and recertification process is governed by the National Board on Certification and Recertification of Nurse Anesthetists (NBCRNA). The NBCRNA exists as an autonomous not-for-profit incorporated organization so as to prevent any conflict of interest with the AANA. This provides assurance to the public that CRNA candidates have met unbiased certification requirements that have exceeded benchmark qualifications and knowledge of anesthesia. CRNAs also have continuing education requirements and recertification check-ins every two years thereafter, plus any additional requirements of the state in which they practice. The new recertification pathway focuses on: maintenance of certification, life long learning, and continued competence. The Continued Professional Certification (CPC) Program consists of 8-year periods, and each period comprises two four-year cycles. In addition to practice and license requirements, the program includes four main components: class A credits, class B credits, core modules, and an examination. Research in the area of maintainance of certification post initial training for medical and nursing specialties is emerging. The CPC program for CRNAs is meant to serve the needs of the public and certificant stakeholders alike and is designed to evolve based on current evidence.

Legal Challenges

In the United States, there have been three challenges brought against nurse anesthetists for illegally practicing medicine: *Frank v. South* in 1917, Hodgins and Crile in 1919, and *Chalmers-Fran-*

cis v. Nelson in 1936. All occurred before 1940 and all were found in favor of the nursing profession, relying on the premise that the surgeon in charge of the operating room was the person practicing medicine. Prior to World War II, the delivery of anesthesia was mainly a nursing function. There were limited anesthetic drug choices and less was known about the physiologic effects of anesthesia and surgery. In 1942, there were 17 nurse anesthetists for every one anesthesiologist. As knowledge grew and surgery became more complex, the numbers of physicians in this specialty expanded in the late 1960s. Therefore, it was legally established that when a nurse delivers anesthesia, it is the practice of nursing. When a physician delivers anesthesia, it is the practice of medicine. When a dentist delivers anesthesia, it is the practice of dentistry. There are great overlaps of tasks in the health care professions. Administration of anesthesia and its related tasks by one provider does not necessarily contravene the practice of other health care providers. For example, endotracheal intubation (placing a breathing tube into the windpipe) is performed by physicians, physician assistants, nurse anesthetists, anesthesiologist assistants, respiratory therapists, paramedics, EMT-Intermediates, and dental (maxillofacial) surgeons. In the United States, nurse anesthetists practice under the state's nursing practice act (not medical practice acts), which outlines the scope of practice for anesthesia nursing.

Scope of Practice

Today, nurse anesthetists practice in all 50 United States and administer approximately 43 million anesthetics each year (AANA). CRNA practice varies from state to state, and is also dependent on the institution in which CRNAs practice.

CRNAs practice in a wide variety of public and private settings including large academic medical centers, small community hospitals, outpatient surgery centers, pain clinics, or physician's offices, either working together with anesthesiologists, other CRNAs, or in independent practice. When practicing within the Anesthesia Care Team model, CRNAs most often fall under the medical direction, or supervision, of an anesthesiologist, although that is not a requirement. CRNAs also have a substantial role in the military, the Veterans Administration (VA), and public health.

The degree of independence or supervision by a licensed provider (physician, dentist, or podiatrist) varies with state law. Some states use the term collaboration to define a relationship where the supervising physician is responsible for the patient and provides medical direction for the nurse anesthetist. Other states require the consent or order of a physician or other qualified licensed provider to administer the anesthetic. No state requires supervision specifically by an anesthesiologist.

The licensed CRNA is authorized to deliver comprehensive anesthesia care under the particular Nurse Practice Act of each state. Their anesthesia practice consists of all accepted anesthetic techniques including general, epidural, spinal, sedation, or local. Scope of CRNA practice is commonly further defined by the practice location's clinical privilege and credentialing process, anesthesia department policies, or practitioner agreements. Clinical privileges are based on the scope and complexity of the expected clinical practice, CRNA qualifications, and CRNA experience. This allows the CRNA to provide core services and activities under defined conditions with or without supervision.

In 2001, the Centers for Medicare and Medicaid Services (CMS) published a rule in the Federal

Register that allows a state to be exempt from Medicare's physician supervision requirement for nurse anesthetists after appropriate approval by the state governor. To date, 17 states have opted out of the federal requirement, instituting their own individual requirements instead.

More than 40 percent of the CRNAs are men, a much greater percentage than in the nursing profession as a whole (ten percent of all nurses are men).

Because many less-developed countries have few anesthesiologists, they rely mainly on nurse anesthetists for anesthesia services. In 1989, the International Federation of Nurse Anesthetists was established. The International Federation of Nurse Anesthetists has since increased in membership and has become a voice for nurse anesthetists worldwide. They have developed standards of education, practice, and a code of ethics. Delegates from 35 member countries participate in the World Congress every few years. Currently there are 107 countries where nurse anesthetists train and practice and nine countries where nurses assist in the administration of anesthesia.

Armed Forces

In the United States armed forces, nurse anesthetists provide a critical peacetime and wartime skill. During peacetime and wartime, nurse anesthetists have been the principal providers of anesthesia services for active duty and retired service members and their dependents. Nurse anesthetists function as the only licensed independent anesthesia practitioners at many military treatment facilities, including U.S. Navy ships at sea. They are also the leading provider of anesthesia for the Veterans Administration and Public Health Service medical facilities.

During World War I, America's nurse anesthetists played a vital role in the care of combat troops in France. From 1914 to 1915, three years prior to America entering the war, Dr. George Crile and nurse anesthetists Agatha Hodgins and Mabel Littleton served in the Lakeside Unit at the American Ambulance at Neuilly-sur-Seine in France. In addition, they helped train the French and British nurses and physicians in anesthesia care. After the war, France continued to use nurse anesthetists; however, Britain adopted a physician-only policy that continues today. In 1917, the American participation in the war resulted in the U.S. military training nurse anesthetists for service. The Army and Navy sent nurses anesthesia trainees to various hospitals, including the Mayo Clinic at Rochester and the Lakeside Hospital in Cleveland before overseas service.

Among notable nurse anesthetists are Sophie Gran Winton. She served with the Red Cross at an army hospital in Château-Thierry, France, and earned the French Croix de Guerre in addition to other service awards. In addition, Anne Penland was the first nurse anesthetist to serve on the British Front and was decorated by the British government.

American nurse anesthetists also served in World War II and Korea, receiving numerous citations and awards. Second Lieutenant Mildred Irene Clark provided anesthesia for casualties from the Japanese attack on Pearl Harbor. During the Vietnam War, nurse anesthetists served as both CRNAs and flight nurses, and also developed new field equipment. Nurse anesthetists have been casualties of war. Lieutenants Kenneth R. Shoemaker, Jr. and Jerome E. Olmsted, were killed in an air evac mission en route to Qui Nhon, Vietnam.

At least one nurse anesthetist was a prisoner of war. Army Nurse anesthetist Annie Mealer endured a three-year imprisonment by the Japanese in the Philippines, and was released in 1945. During the Iraq War, nurse anesthetists comprise the largest group of anesthesia providers at forward positioned medical treatment facilities. In addition, they play a role in the continuing education and training of Department of Defense nurses and technicians in the care of wartime trauma patients.

Certified Nurse Midwife

In the United States, a certified nurse midwife (CNM) is an advanced practice registered nurse in nurse midwifery, the care of women across their lifespan, including pregnancy and the postpartum period, and well woman care and birth control. Certified nurse midwives are exceptionally recognized by the International Confederation of Midwives as a type of midwives in the United States.

Education and Training

The American College of Nurse-Midwives accredits certified nurse-midwifery education programs and serves as the national specialty society for the nation's CNMs. CNMs in most states are required to

- possess a minimum of a graduate degree, such as the Master of Science in Nursing or a Doctorate of Nursing Practice.

- pass the NCLEX examination to become a registered nurse.

- pass the American Midwifery Certification Board exams.

- hold an active registered nurse license in the state in which they practice.

- keep up to date on latest medical knowledge as pertains to their field.

In 2010 the first wave of CNMs graduated from Doctor of Nursing Practice (DNP) programs. The American College of Nurse-Midwives (ACNM) estimates that soon, one in ten babies in the U.S. will be delivered by CNMs. In 2010 the first DNP program available for CNMs graduated its first class.

Practice

CNMs function as primary healthcare providers for women and most often provide medical care for relatively healthy women, whose health and births are considered uncomplicated and not "high risk," as well as their neonates. Often, women with high risk pregnancies can receive the benefits of nurse midwifery care from a CNM in collaboration with a physician. CNMs may work closely or in collaboration, with an obstetrician & gynecologist, who provides consultation and/or assistance to patients who develop complications or have complex medical histories or disease(s). CNMs provide health care for sexual health, as they also see women for routine exams and are able to initiate all types of contraception.

CNMs practice in hospitals and private practice medical clinics and may also deliver babies in birthing centers and attend at-home births. Some work with academic institutions as professors.

They are able to prescribe medications, treatments, medical devices, therapeutic and diagnostic measures. CNMs are able to provide medical care to women from puberty through menopause, including care for their newborn (neonatology), antepartum, intrapartum, postpartum and nonsurgical gynecological care. In some cases, CNMs may also provide care to the male partner, in areas of sexually transmitted diseases and reproductive health, of their female patients. In the United States, fewer than 1% of nurse midwives are men.

Clinical Nurse Specialist

A clinical nurse specialist (CNS) is an advanced practice nurse who can provide expert advice related to specific conditions or treatment pathways. According to the International Council of Nurses (ICN), an Advanced Practice Nurse is a registered nurse who has acquired the expert knowledge base, complex decision-making skills and clinical competencies for expanded practice, the characteristics of which are shaped by the context and/or country in which s/he is credentialed to practice. Clinical Nurse Specialists are registered nurses, who have graduate level nursing preparation at the master's or doctoral level as a CNS. They are clinical experts in evidence-based nursing practice within a specialty area, treating and managing the health concerns of patients and populations. The CNS specialty may be focused on individuals, populations, settings, type of care, type of problem, or diagnostic systems subspecialty. CNSs practice autonomously and integrate knowledge of disease and medical treatments into the assessment, diagnosis, and treatment of patients' illnesses. These nurses design, implement, and evaluate both patient–specific and population-based programs of care. CNSs provide leadership in the advanced practice of nursing to achieve quality and cost-effective patient outcomes as well as provide leadership of multidisciplinary groups in designing and implementing innovative alternative solutions that address system problems and/or patient care issues. In many jurisdictions, CNSs, as direct care providers, perform comprehensive health assessments, develop differential diagnoses, and may have prescriptive authority. Prescriptive authority allows them to provide pharmacologic and nonpharmacologic treatments and order diagnostic and laboratory tests in addressing and managing specialty health problems of patients and populations. CNSs serve as patient advocates, consultants, and researchers in various settings [American Nurses Association (ANA) Scope and Standards of Practice (2004), p. 15].

United States

In the United States a CNS is an advanced practice registered nurse (APRN), with graduate preparation (earned master's or doctorate) from a program that prepares CNSs. The National Association of Clinical Nurse Specialists (NACNS) announced in July 2015 its endorsement of proposals for the Doctor of Nursing Practice (DNP) as the required degree for CNS entry into practice by 2030. According to the Consensus Model for APRN Regulation (2008), "The CNS has a unique APRN role to integrate care across the continuum and through three spheres of influence: patient, nurse, system. The three spheres are overlapping and interrelated but each sphere possesses a distinctive focus. In each of the spheres of influence, the primary goal of the CNS is continuous improvement of patient outcomes and nursing care. Key elements of CNS practice are to create environments through mentoring and (p. 8) system changes that empower nurses to develop caring, evidence-based practices to alleviate patient distress, facilitate ethical decision-making, and respond to diversity. The CNS is responsible and accountable for diagnosis and treatment of health/ illness states, disease management, health promotion, and prevention of illness and risk behaviors among individuals, families, groups, and communities." (p. 9). CNSs are clinical experts in a specialized area of nursing practice and in the delivery of evidence-based nursing interventions.

A systematic review published in 2011 identified 11 studies from the US (four RCTs and seven observational) that had looked at the possible effect of having CNS as part of the healthcare team. The reviewers found some evidence of reduced length of stay and costs of care for teams which included a CNS.

Overview

CNSs work with other nurses to advance their nursing practices, improve outcomes, and provide clinical expertise to effect system-wide changes to improve programs of care. CNSs work in specialties that are defined by one of the following categories:

- Population (e.g. pediatrics, geriatrics, women's health)

- Setting (e.g. critical care, emergency department, long-term care)

- Disease or Medical Subspecialty (e.g. diabetes, oncology, palliative)

- Type of Care (e.g. psychiatric, rehabilitation)

- Type of Problem (e.g. pain, wounds, palliative)

Spheres of Influence

There are three domains of CNS practice, known as the *three spheres of influence* (NACNS 2004):

- Patient

- Nursing personnel

- System (healthcare system)

The three spheres are overlapping and interrelated, but each sphere possesses a distinctive focus. In each of the spheres of influence, the primary goal of the CNS is continuous improvement of patient outcomes and nursing care.

Core Competencies

Within the three spheres of CNS practice, Sparacino (2005) identified seven core competencies:

1. Direct clinical practice includes expertise in advanced assessment, implementing nursing care, and evaluating outcomes.

2. Expert coaching and guidance encompasses modeling clinical expertise while helping nurses integrate new evidence into practice. It also means providing education or teaching skills to patients and family.

3. Collaboration focuses on multidisciplinary team building.

4. Consultation involves reviewing alternative approaches and implementing planned change.

5. Research involves interpreting and using research, evaluating practice, and collaborating in research.

6. Clinical and professional leadership involves responsibility for innovation and change in the patient care system.

7. Ethical decision-making involves influence in negotiating moral dilemmas, allocating resources, directing patient care and access to care.

Although these core competencies have been described in the literature they are not validated through a review process that is objective and decisive. They are the opinion of some within the profession. A set of core competencies has now been described and validated through a consensus process (2008) that clearly defines the spheres of influence, the synergy model and the competencies as defined by Sparacino (2005). These core competencies are now expected to be used in all educational programs and will be revised in the coming years in order to be maintained as current and reflective of practice. The 2010 Adult-Gerontology Clinical Nurse Specialist Core Competencies revision reflect the work of a national Expert Panel, representing the array of both adult and gerontology clinical nurse specialist education and practice. In collaboration with colleagues from the Hartford Geriatric Nursing Institute at New York University and the National Association of Clinical Nurse Specialists (NACNS), the American Association of Colleges of Nursing (AACN) facilitated the process to develop these consensus-based competencies, including the work of the national Expert Panel and the external validation process. Pivotal to the full practice authority of CNSs in the United States as intended by the APRN Consensus Model implementation is the inclusion in the core competencies of the Clinical Nurse Specialists the crucial role of prescribing medications and durable medical equipment. The authoritative 2010 CNS core competencies document states that the clinical nurse specialist prescribes nursing therapeutics, pharmacologic and non-pharmacologic interventions, diagnostic measures, equipment, procedures, and treatments to meet the needs of patients, families and groups, in accordance with professional preparation, institutional privileges, state and federal laws and practice acts.

International Perspectives

Historically, in North America, the CNS role developed within the acute care (hospital) setting. Currently, in addition to the traditional acute care setting, CNSs practice in a variety of non-acute care settings.

In the Australian Health System, however, a clinical nurse specialist refers to a promotional position, rather than a qualification.

Nurse Practitioner

Nurse practitioners are advanced registered nurses educated and trained to provide health promotion and maintenance through the diagnosis and treatment of acute illness and chronic condition.

According to the International Council of Nurses, an advanced practice registered nurse (APRN) is "a registered nurse who has acquired the expert knowledge base, complex decision-making skills and clinical competencies for expanded practice, the characteristics of which are shaped by the context and/or country in which s/he is credentialed to practice. A master's degree is recommended for entry level."

Overview

Nurse practitioners (NPs) manage acute and chronic medical conditions, both physical and mental, through history and physical exam and the ordering of diagnostic tests and medical treatments. NPs are qualified to diagnose medical problems, order treatments, perform advanced procedures, prescribe medications, and make referrals for a wide range of acute and chronic medical conditions within their scope of practice. Nurse Practitioners have become such an integral part of the medical and health care system. This is all in part to the combination of experience and expertise they bring with them. The experience from working as a nurse gives them a unique approach in providing patient care, while their advanced studies give them the expertise and capability to carry on tasks otherwise assigned to physicians. NPs work in hospitals, private offices, clinics, and nursing homes/long term care facilities. Some nurse practitioners contract out their services for private duty.

In the United States, depending upon the state in which they work, nurse practitioners may or may not be required to practice under the supervision of a physician. In consideration of the shortage of primary care/internal medicine physicians, many states are eliminating "collaborative practice" agreements and nurse practitioners are able to function independently. NPs—particularly in the area of primary care/internal medicine—fulfill a vital need for patient healthcare services, and the nurse practitioner works with physicians, medical/surgical specialists, pharmacists, physical therapists, social workers, occupational therapists, and other healthcare professionals to achieve the best outcomes for patients.

NPs may serve as a patient's primary healthcare provider and they may treat patients of all ages depending upon their specialty. With commensurate education and experience, nurse practitioners may specialize in areas such as cardiology, dermatology, oncology, pain management, surgical services, orthopedics, women's health, and other specialties. Similar to all healthcare professions, the core philosophy of the nurse practitioner role is individualized care that focuses on a patient's medical issues as well as the effects of illness on the life of a patient and his or her family. NPs tend to concentrate on a holistic approach to patient care, and they emphasize health promotion, patient education/counseling, and disease prevention. The main classifications of nurse practitioners are: adult (ANP); acute care (ACNP); gerontological (GNP); family (FNP); pediatric (PNP); neonatal (NNP); and psychiatric-mental health (PMHNP). Adult-gerontology primary care nurse practitioner (AGPCNP) is a classification that has recently evolved.

In addition to providing a wide range of healthcare services, nurse practitioners may conduct research, teach, and are often active in patient advocacy and in the development of healthcare policy at the local, state, and national level.

History

The advanced practice nursing role began to take shape in the mid-20th century United States. Nurse anesthetists and nurse midwives were established in the 1940s, followed by psychiatric nursing in 1954. The present day concept of the APRN as a primary care provider was created in the mid-1960s, spurred on by a national shortage of medical doctors. The first formal graduate certificate program for nurse practitioners was created by Henry Silver, a physician, and Loretta Ford, a nurse, in 1965, with a vision to help balance rising healthcare costs, increase the number of healthcare providers, and correct the inefficient distribution of health resources. In 1971, The U.S. Secretary of Health, Education and Welfare, Elliot Richardson, made a formal recommendation in expanding the scope of the nursing practice and qualifying them to be able to serve as primary care providers. During the mid 1970s to early 1980s, the completion of a master's degree became required in order to become a certified nurse practitioner. In 2012, discussions have risen between accreditation agencies, national certifying bodies, and state boards of nursing about the possibility of making the DNP as the new minimum of education for NP certification and licensure by 2015.

Scope of Practice

United States

In the United States, because the profession is state-regulated, care provided by NPs varies and is limited to their education and credentials. Some NPs seek to work independently of physicians, while in some states a collaborative agreement with a physician is required for practice. The extent of this collaborative agreement, and the role, duties, responsibilities, nursing treatments, pharmacologic recommendations, etc. again varies widely amongst states of licensure/certification.

The "Pearson Report" provides a current state-by-state breakdown of the specific duties an NP may perform in the state. A nurse practitioner's role may include the following:

- Medical diagnosis, treatment, evaluation, and management of a wide range of acute and chronic diseases

- Obtaining patient histories and conducting physical examinations

- Requesting diagnostic imaging

- Performing some diagnostic studies (e.g., lab tests and EKGs)

- Requesting physical therapy, occupational therapy, and other rehabilitation treatments

- Prescribing drugs for acute and chronic illness (extent of prescriptive authority varies by state regulations)

- Providing prenatal care and family planning services

- Providing well-child care, including screening and immunizations

- Providing primary and specialty care services, health-maintenance care for adults, including annual physicals

- Providing care for patients in acute and critical care settings and long care facilities

- Performing or assisting in minor surgeries and procedures (e.g., dermatological biopsies/procedures, suturing, casting, etc.)

- Counseling and educating patients on health behaviors, self-care skills, and treatment options in coordination with occupational therapists and other healthcare providers.

Canada

In Canada, an NP is a registered nurse with a graduate degree in nursing. Canada recognizes them in the following specialties: primary healthcare NPs (PHCNP) and acute care NPs (ACNP). NP's diagnose illnesses, prescribe pharmaceuticals, order and interpret diagnostic tests, and perform procedures in their scope of practice. PHCNPs work in places like community healthcare centers, primary healthcare settings and long term care institutions. The main focus of PHCNPs includes health promotion, preventative care, treatment and diagnosis of acute illnesses and injuries, and overseeing and managing chronic diseases. ANCNPs are specialized NPs who serve a specific population of patients. They administer care to individuals who are acutely, critically or chronically ill patients. ANCNPs generally work in in-patient facilities that include neonatology, nephrology, and cardiology units.

Range of Practice

United States

Nurse Practitioner's can examine patients, diagnose illnesses, prescribe medication, and provide treatments. These are all responsibilities that entail physicians but NP's do not have the authority of all physicians in all 50 states. Less than half of the country permits NP's the authority to practice on their own. In fact, only 20 states (including D.C.) give full practice authority to NP's. Nineteen states require NP's to have a written agreement with a physician in order to provide care. Even with the formal agreement between physican and NP's, their practice is restricted in at least one domain (e.g., prescribing, treatment). The remaining 12 states restrict NP's even more. In order for NP's to provide care to patients, they are required to be supervised or delegated by a physician. The states in the Pacific Northwest, the Mountain states, and in upper New England generally have fewer and limited primary care physicians so they permit more freedom to NP's. Many states in the South are the most restrictive states.

Education, Licensing, and Board Certification

United States

The path to becoming a nurse practitioner in the United States begins by earning a Bachelor of Science in Nursing (BSN) or other undergraduate degree, and requires licensure as a registered nurse (RN) and experience in the generalist RN role. Then, one must graduate from an accredited graduate (MSN) or doctoral (DNP) program. The typical curriculum for a nurse practitioner program includes courses in epidemiology; health promotion; advanced pathophysiology; physical assessment and diagnostic reasoning; advanced pharmacology; laboratory/radiography diagnostics; statistics and research methods; health policy; role development and leadership; acute and chronic disease management (e.g., adults, children, women's health, geriatrics, etc.); and clinical rotations, which varies depending on the program and population focus. Doctor of Nursing Practice (DNP) programs include additional, advanced coursework in biostatistics; research methods; clinical outcome measures; care of special populations; organizational management; informatics;

and healthcare policy and economics. DNP programs also require completion of a research project/residency. Some nurse practitioners, as well as other APRN roles, may choose to pursue the Doctor of Philosophy (PhD) as a terminal degree. The PhD in nursing focuses on nursing research and nursing education, while the DNP focuses more on clinical practice.

There is an initiative to require the DNP as the entry level degree for all APRN roles, including the nurse practitioner, nurse anesthetist, clinical nurse specialist, and nurse midwife. Those who have a MSN but are currently practicing in an APRN role would be grandfathered into this change. Many universities have started to phase out MSN programs in lieu of this expected change and have devised BSN-DNP programs. NPs may elect to complete a postgraduate residency or fellowship. The majority of such programs focus on primary care; however, specialized programs (e.g., acute care, emergency medicine, cardiology, general surgery, etc.) also exist.

After completing the required education, the NP must pass a national board certifying exam in a specific population focus: acute care, family practice, women's health, pediatrics, adult-gerontology, neonatal, or psychiatric-mental health, which coincides with the type of program from which he or she graduated. After achieving board certification, the nurse practitioners must apply for additional credentials (e.g., APRN license, prescriptive authority, DEA registration number, etc.) at the state and federal level. The nurse practitioner must achieve a certain amount of continuing medical education (CME) credits and clinical practice hours in order to maintain certification and licensure. NPs are licensed through state boards of nursing.

Australia

In Australia, NPs are required to be registered by the Australian Health Practitioner Regulation Agency. The Australian professional organisation is the Australian College of Nurse Practitioners. (ACNP)

Canada

In Canada, the educational standard is a graduate degree in nursing. The Canadian Nursing Association (CNA) notes that advanced practice nurses must have a combination of a graduate level education and the clinical experience that prepare them to practice at an advanced level. Their education alone does not give them the ability to practice at an advanced level. Two national frameworks have been developed in order to provide further guidance for the development of educational courses and requirements, research concepts, and government position statements regarding APRNs: The CNA's *Advanced Nursing Practice: A National Framework* and the *Canadian Nurse Practitioner Core Competency Framework*. All educational programs for NPs must achieve formal approval by provincial and territorial regulating nurse agencies due to the fact that the NP is considered a legislated role in Canada. As such, it is common to see differences among approved educational programs between territories and provinces. Specifically, inconsistencies can be found in core graduate courses, clinical experiences, and length of programs. Canada does not have a national curriculum or consistent standards regarding advanced practice nurses so all APRNs must meet individual requirements set by the provincial or territorial regulatory nursing body where they are practicing. In conclusion, the completion of a graduate education, a passing of an exam through the CNA Nurse Practitioner Exam Program, and a successful registration within the appropriate territory or province is required in order to practice as a nurse practitioner in Canada.

Other Countries

There are nurse practitioners in over fifty countries worldwide. Although credentials vary by country, most NPs hold at least a master's degree worldwide.

As of November 2013, NPs were recognized legally in Israel. The law passed on November 21, 2013. Although in the early stages, the Israeli Ministry of Health has already graduated two NP classes - in palliative care and geriatrics. The law was passed in response to a growing physician shortage in specific health care fields, similar to trends occurring worldwide.

Nurse Practitioner titles were in the past bestowed on some advanced practice registered nurses in the Netherlands. The title has now changed to that of *Nursing Specialist*. The idea is still the same: a master's-degree-level independently licensed nurse capable of setting indications for treatment independent of an MD.

Salary

The salary of a nurse practitioner depends on the area of specialization, location, years of experience, level of education, and size of company. In 2015 the American Academy of Nurse Practitioners (AANP) conducted it's 4th annual nurse practitioner salary survey. The results revealed the salary range of a NP to be between $98,760 to $108,643 reported income among full-time NPs. According to the U.S. Bureau of Labor Statistics, nurse practitioners in the top 10% earned an average salary of $135,800. The median salary was $98,190. According to a report published by Merritt Hawkins, starting salaries for NPs increased in dramatic fashion between 2015 and 2016. The highest average starting salary reached $197,000 in 2016. The primary factor in the dramatic increase in starting salaries is skyrocketing demand for NPs, recognizing them as the 5th most highly sought after advanced health professional in 2016.

Increasing Need in US

Employment of registered nurses and nurse practitioners is expected to increase immensely in the next ten years. Much of the growth is expected to come as a result of advances in technology, leading to better health care and a greater variety of solutions for health problems. Also, life expectancy is getting longer; therefore more patients are living longer and living more active lives. It is further anticipated that the need for NPs will increase because of the passage of the Patient Protection and Affordable Care Act (PPACA).

Growth is also expected to be much faster in outpatient centers, where the patients do not stay overnight. Moreover, the increasing number of procedures that were once only able to happen in hospitals is now able to happen in physicians' offices. That is mainly because of the expansion and easy access to new and better technology, but the need for NPs is expected to be greatest in places where people have long-term illnesses such as dementia or head trauma patients that are in need of extensive rehabilitation.

"Nurse practitioners really are becoming a growing presence, particularly in primary care," said David I. Auerbach, PhD, the author and a health economist at RAND Corp. In addition, this site says that nurse practitioners are expected to double by 2025. Auerbach also told *American Medi-*

cal News, "There's a lot of experimentation going on looking at different ways of working together, and there's a lot of interest in collaborative team-based models. The new care models, such as the patient-centered medical home and accountable care organizations, really depend on nurse practitioners and physician assistants."

As a result of the PPACA, hospitals and medical care facilities are forced to rethink the demand for nurses and medical professionals. This is mainly because this new Act allows millions of people the opportunity at medical attention that did not have it before, and because there are so many new people in need of medical attention, the need for medical professionals also grows. With the combination of this new Act, and the aging Baby Boomer population, there is expected to be a large increase in the need for medical staff, especially nurse practitioners. According to a study published in American Medical News, Nurse Practitioners jobs are expected to grow up to 130 percent from 86,000 in 2008 to 198,000 in 2025. Though there is some skepticism to these vast figures, they are backed up by many studies and the opinions of very well known medical professionals. As a result of this extreme need for NPs, they are also expected to receive more autonomy, meaning that nurse practitioners would be able to fill the traditional primary care role like a physician would. For an example, a nurse practitioner would be able to prescribe medication without the oversight of a doctor. Many states are passing laws that allow for independent practice of nurse practitioners. "Currently there are 12 states with active legislation looking at utilizing nurse practitioners at the top of their education to meet patient care needs," says Tay Kopanos with the American Association of Nurse Practitioners. Many nurses and other leaders in healthcare are advocating for overturning laws that require physicians to look over the work of NPs.

Emergency Nursing

Emergency nursing is a specialty within the field of professional nursing focusing on the care of patients with medical emergencies, that is, those who require prompt medical attention to avoid long-term disability or death. Emergency nurses are most frequently employed in hospital emergency departments (EDs), although they may also work in urgent care centers, sports arenas, and on medical transport helicopters and ambulances.

ED Nurse Role

In addition to addressing these "true emergencies," emergency nurses increasingly care for people who are unwilling or unable to get primary medical care elsewhere and come to emergency departments for help.

Besides heart attacks, strokes, gunshot wounds and car accidents, emergency nurses also tend to patients with acute alcohol and/or drug intoxication, psychiatric and behavioral problems and those who have been raped.

They must be adept at working with patients of many different backgrounds, cultures, religions, ages and types of disabilities. Emergency nurses must also have a good working knowledge of the many legal issues impacting health care such as consent, handling of evidence, mandatory reporting of child and elder abuse and involuntary psychiatric holds.

In their role as patient educators, they must have a thorough knowledge of anatomy, physiology, pharmacology and psychology and be able to communicate effectively with patients and their families.

An emergency nurse is typically assigned to triage patients as they arrive in the emergency department and as such are the first professional patients see. Therefore, the emergency nurse must be skilled at rapid, accurate physical examination, early recognition of life-threatening conditions. In some cases, emergency nurses may order certain tests and medications following "collaborative practice guidelines" or "standing orders" set out by the hospital's emergency physician staff.

Board Certification in Emergency Nursing

CEN®

The Certified Emergency Nurse (CEN)® designation is granted to a registered nurse who has demonstrated expertise in emergency nursing by passing a computer-administered examination given by the Board of Certification for Emergency Nursing (BCEN). The certification exam first became available in July 1980, was accredited by ABSNC in February 2002, and was reaccredited in 2007 and 2012. The certification is valid for four years, and can be renewed either by passing another examination, by completing 100 continuing education units (CEUs) in the specialty, or by completing an online 150 question "open book exam."

As of 2015, the BCEN has designated over 30,500 active CENs in the United States and Canada. The CEN exam has 175 questions; 150 are used for testing purposes (25 are sample questions). The passing score is 70% and the candidate has three hours to take the exam. The test is administered internationally in Pearson Vue testing centers.

CPEN®

The Certified Pediatric Emergency Nurse (CPEN)® designation is applied to a registered nurse who has demonstrated expertise in pediatric emergency nursing by passing a computer-administered examination given jointly by the Board of Certification for Emergency Nursing (BCEN) and the Pediatric Nursing Certification Board (PNCB). The certification exam first became available on January 21, 2009, and was accredited by ABSNC in May 2015. The certification is valid for four years, and can be renewed either by passing another examination, by completing 100 contact hours (continuing education) in the specialty, or by completing 1,000 clinical practice hours and 40 contact hours in the specialty. The CPEN exam has 175 questions; 25 are unscored sample questions.

As of 2015, the BCEN and the PNCB have designated over 3,900 active CPENs. The CPEN exam has 175 questions; 150 are used for testing purposes (25 are sample questions). The passing score is 87% and the candidate has three hours to take the exam. The test is administered in AMP testing centers internationally.

Emergency Nurse Practitioner (ENP)

In the United Kingdom

A specialist nurse will independently assess, diagnose, investigate, and treat a wide range of common accidents and injuries working autonomously without reference to medical staff. They primarily treat a wide range of musculoskeletal problems, skin problems and minor illnesses. They are trained in advanced nursing skills. Under the National Health Service grading system, ENPs are typically graded Band 6 or 7.

Additionally, some specialized nurses perform as [emergency care practitioner]s. They generally work in the pre-hospital setting dealing with a wide range of medical or emergency problems. Their primary function is to assess, diagnose and treat a patient in the home in an emergency setting.

In the United States

An advanced practice nurse assesses, diagnoses, and treats a variety of common illnesses, injuries and disease processes in emergency care settings. ENPs are trained in advanced nursing and medical skills such as x-ray interpretation, ophthalmic slit lamp examination, suturing, local and regional anesthesia, abscess incision and drainage, advanced airway techniques, fracture reduction, and casting and splinting.

In Australia

Australian nurse practitioners follow the clinical practice guidelines developed by the Victorian Emergency Nurse Practitioner Collaborative (VENPC), who have supported nurse practitioner development in Victoria. This includes attending to minor head injuries, burns, open wounds, joint pain (Haemophilia), blood and fluid exposure, PV bleeding, suspected UTI, abdominal pain, cellulitis and more.

Challenges of Emergency Nursing

Emergency nursing is a demanding job and can be unpredictable. Emergency nurses need to have basic knowledge of most specialty areas, to be able to work under pressure, communicate effectively with many types of patients, collaborate with a variety of health care providers and prioritize the tasks that must be performed.

It can be quite draining both physically and mentally for many nurses. Australian emergency department treat over 7 million patients each year. They spend much of their time on their feet and ready for unexpected changes in patients' conditions as well as sudden influxes of patients to the emergency department. ED (emergency department) nurses may be exposed to traumatic situations such as heavy bleeding, dismemberment and even death.

Violence is a growing challenge for many nurses in the ED. Emergency nurses too often receive both physical and verbal abuse from patients and visitors.

Emergency Nurses in Africa

Emergency nurses work in various places, many of which are understaffed as there are nursing shortages across Africa. There is also a shortage of doctors, leaving many tasks for nurses with limited guidelines or standards to deal with, and for many emergency nurses the scope of practice is quite undefined. Nurses may be forced to work outside their scope causing frustration and increasing the opportunities for occupational health hazards. It can be speculated that triage protocols are either lacking or not being followed. The limited basic knowledge and skill of emergency nursing included in undergraduate nurse training programs, and the limited number of nurse trainers, provide difficulty for many pending nurses to acquire the skills needed to work in emergency settings.

The History of Emergency Nursing

Around the 1800s hospitals became more popular and there was a growth in emergency care. The first development of an emergency room was originally called "The First Aid Room". Originally, nurses only dressed wounds, applied eye ointments, treated minor burns with salves and bandages, and attended patients with minor illnesses like colds and sore throats. The rule of thumb was first in, first served, but there were many cases where some people were in more need of emergency care than others and as the situation became more intolerable, one of the greatest medical developments came into perspective: triage.

For centuries triage had been used in war but was not yet established in the emergency department. The first time triage was referred to during a non-disaster issue was at Yale, Newhaven Hospital, United States, in 1963, and since then has become developed and more defined.

Additional Emergency Nursing Education/certification

- Advanced Burn Life Support (ABLS)

- Advanced Cardiac Life Support (ACLS)

- Advanced Medical Life Support (AMLS)

- Advanced Trauma Care for Nurses (ATCN)

- Basic Life Support (BLS)

- Course in Advanced Trauma (CATN)

- Emergency Nursing Pediatric Course (ENPC)

- Geriatric Emergency Nursing Education (GENE)

- Mobile Intensive Care Nurse (MICN)

- National Institutes of Health Stroke Scale Certification (NIHSS)

- Neonatal Resuscitation Program (NRP)

- Pediatric Advanced Life Support (PALS)

- Pre-Hospital Emergency Care (PHEC)

- Trauma Nursing Core Course (TNCC)

References

- Mitchell, L; Flin, R (2008). "Non-technical skills of the operating theatre scrub nurse: Literature review". Journal of Advanced Nursing. 63 (1): 15–24. doi:10.1111/j.1365-2648.2008.04695

- Hamlin, L; Davies, M; Richardson-Tench, M (2011). Perioperative Nursing: An introductory text. Elsevier Health Sciences APAC. pp. chapter 12, 293–295. ISBN 9780729538879

- "Welch Allyn Connex Clinical Surveillance System for Continuous Multiple Parameter Patient Monitoring". Medgadget. 2014-02-13. Retrieved 2016-05-17

- "Surgical nurses' different understandings of their interactions with patients: A phenomenographic study". Scandinavian Journal of Caring Sciences. 25 (3): 533–541. 2011. doi:10.1111/j.1471-6712.2010.00860

- Rooks, Judith Pence (1997). Midwifery and childbirth in America. Philadelphia: Temple University Press. p. 422. ISBN 1-56639-711-1

- Hutcherson, Carolyn M (September 30, 2001). "Legal Considerations for Nurses Practicing in a Telehealth Setting". Online Journal of Issues in Nursing. 6 (3). Retrieved 12 May 2016

- "Angels of the Airfields: Navy Air Evacuation Nurses of World War II | Naval Historical Foundation". www.navyhistory.org. Retrieved 2016-05-18

- Institut Européen des Sciences de la Santé. "Licence en Sciences Infirmières - Soins Oncologiques". IESS Maroc. Retrieved 1 August 2014

- Tse, K; So, W.K. (2008). "Nurses' perceptions of preoperative teaching for ambulatory surgical patients". Journal of Advanced Nursing. 63 (6): 619–625. doi:10.1111/j.1365-2648.2008.04744

- Leavitt, Judith W. (1988). Brought to Bed: Childbearing in America, 1750-1950. Book: Oxford University Press. p. 178. ISBN 978-0195056907

- American Association of Nurse Anesthetists (1995). "AANA Archives: Documenting a distinguished past." Retrieved December 28

- Van Teijlingen, Edwin R.; Lowis, George W.; McCaffery, Peter G. (2004). Midwifery and the Medicalization of Childbirth: Comparative Perspectives. Nova Publishers. ISBN 9781594540318

- American Association of Nurse Anesthetists (2007)Scope and Standards for Nurse Anesthesia Practice. Retrieved May 24, 2007

- Brideson, G (2015). "Images of flight nursing in Australia: A study using institutional ethnography". Nursing and Health Sciences. doi:10.1111/nhs.12225

- Borst, Charlotte G. (1995). Catching Babies: The Professionalization of Childbirth, 1870-1920. Harvard University Press. ISBN 9780674102620

- Halperin, Ofra (2011). "Stressful childbirth situations: A qualitative study of midwives". Journal of Midwifery and Women's Health. doi:10.1111/j.1542-2011.2011.00030

- "Exploring the Spectrum". Maryville University St. Louis Online Nurse Practitioner Programs. Retrieved 24 September 2014

- Ehrenreich, Barbara; Deirdre English (2010). Witches, Midwives and Nurses: A History of Women Healers (2nd ed.). The Feminist Press. pp. 85–87. ISBN 0-912670-13-4

- Hoyt, K. Sue; Proehl, Jean A. (2012). "Affordable Care Act: implications for APRNs". Advanced Emergency Nursing Journal. 34 (4): 287–9. doi:10.1097/TME.0b013e3182729830. PMID 23111302

- "Prenatal care in your first trimester". U.S. Department of Health & Human Services. 1 July 1015. Retrieved 8 August 2015

4

Nursing Management

The management of the employment of nurses is known as nursing management. Some of the processes included in nursing management are organizing, directing, staffing and controlling. Nurse licensure, nurse uniform, nurse-led clinic and nurse–client relationship are the topics explained in the chapter. The aspects elucidated in this chapter are of vital importance, and provide a better understanding of nursing management.

Nursing Management

Nursing management consists of the performance of the leadership functions of governance and decision-making within organizations employing nurses. It includes processes common to all management like planning, organizing, staffing, directing and controlling. It is common for registered nurses to seek additional education to earn a Master of Science in Nursing or Doctor of Nursing Practice to prepare for leadership roles within nursing. Management positions increasingly require candidates to hold an advanced degree in nursing.

Roles

Head of the Nursing Staff

The chief nurse, in other words the person in charge of nursing in a hospital and the head of the nursing staff, is called *nursing officer* in UK English, and *head nurse* or *director of nursing* in US English, and *matron* or *nursing superintendent* in Indian English.

The chief nurse is a registered nurse who supervises the care of all the patients at a health care facility. The chief nurse is the senior nursing management position in an organization and often holds executive titles like *chief nursing officer* (*CNO*), *chief nurse executive*, or *vice-president of nursing*. They typically report to the CEO or COO.

The chief nurse serves as "the head of the general staff of the hospital" and is obeyed by his/her subordinate nurses. Traditionally, chief nurses were called *matrons* and wore a dark-blue dress that was usually darker than that of her subordinates, who were also known as *sisters*, in addition to a white-starched hat. As such, matrons usually "provide strong leadership and act as a link between Board-level nurses and clinical practice." In military hospitals of the United States, matrons were "charged with the responsibility of making twice daily rounds to supervise the [common] nurses' duty performance."

The American Organization of Nurse Executives is a professional association for directors of nursing.

Service Directors

Many large healthcare organizations also have *service directors*. These directors have oversight of a particular service within the facility or system (surgical services, women's services, emergency services, critical care services, etc.).

Nurse manager

The *nurse manager* is the nurse with management responsibilities of a nursing unit. They typically report to a service director. They have primary responsibilities for staffing, budgeting, and day-to-day operations of the unit.

Charge Nurse

The charge nurse is the nurse, usually assigned for a shift, who is responsible for the immediate functioning of the unit. The charge nurse is responsible for making sure nursing care is delivered safely and that all the patients on the unit are receiving adequate care. They are typically the front-line management in most nursing units. Some charge nurses are permanent members of the nursing management team and are called shift supervisors. The traditional term for a female charge nurse is a nursing sister (or just sister), and this term is still commonly used in some countries (such as the United Kingdom and some Commonwealth countries).

Nurse Licensure

Nurse licensure is the process by which various regulatory bodies, usually a Board of Nursing, regulate the practice of nursing within its jurisdiction. The primary purpose of nurse licensure is to grant permission to practice as a nurse after verifying the applicant has met minimal competencies to safely perform nursing activities within nursing's scope of practice. Licensure is necessary when the regulated activities are complex, require specialized knowledge and skill and independent decision making.

Nurse licensure also provides:

- Nursing activities may only be legally performed by individuals holding a nursing license issued by the regulatory body

- Title protection: only the persons issued a license are legally permitted to use certain titles, such as registered nurse, advanced practice registered nurse, etc.

- In order to assure that the public is protected, authority is granted to the regulatory body to take disciplinary action in the event the licensee violate the law or any rules promulgated by the regulatory body

Nurse licensure also establishes a registry of licensed nurses, hence the term "Registered Nurse".

The first nurse licensure and registration program was initiated in 1901 in New Zealand when the Nurses Registration Act 1901 was enacted into law. The first licensure laws in the United States came in 1903. In the US, applicants must successfully pass the NCLEX exam prior to being granted a license.

Director of Nursing (Long-term Care Facility)

A director of nursing (DON) is a registered nurse who supervises the care of all the patients at a health care facility. The director of nursing has special training beyond the training of a staff nurse for the position that pertains to health care management, and in some places, a director of nursing must hold a special license in order to be employed in that capacity.

The director of nursing is one of up to seven directors at a typical health care facility. The other are the directors of food (or dietary) services, social work, activities, business management, house-keeping/laundry, and maintenance. In most facilities, the director of nursing is only second to the facility's administrator, and will fill in in the administrator's absence.

In some facilities, there is also an assistant director of nursing (ADON) who backs up the director of nursing, especially in the DON's absence or off-hours.

The director of nursing is the one who is responsible for communicating between the nursing staff and the physicians at a health care facility. It is the director of nursing who communicates to physicians the needs of the patients.

The director of nursing has the duty of testifying in any criminal or civil legal cases that arise out of the nursing care at the facility and can be held legally liable in the event that his/her own negligence in practice was responsible for a mishap at a facility resulting in death or personal injury to a patient.

Laws Relating to the Director of Nursing

United States

In the United States, federal OBRA regulations set the requirements for directors of nursing.

The director of nursing is a full-time position. Either one person can work in this position for 35 hours in a week, or two or more registered nurses can fulfill the duties for a combined 40 hours in a week.

Duties

The duties of a director of nursing may be as follows:

- Development and implementation of nursing policy and procedure. These must be aimed at preventing accidents at the facility.

- Overseeing the hiring and continued employment of nursing staff

- Ensuring there is adequate nursing staff, and that the staff's skills remain current

- Overseeing nursing employee conduct

- Being a witness at a trial in the event of litigation

- Being knowledgeable of incidents at the facility

- Assessing the health needs of each resident

- Communicating the needs of the residents of the facility to the physicians

Legal Nurse Consultant

A legal nurse consultant (LNC) is a registered nurse who uses expertise as a health care provider and specialized training to consult on medical-related legal cases. LNCs assist attorneys in reading medical records and understanding medical terminology and healthcare issues to achieve the best results for their clients. The specialty is a relatively recent one, beginning in the mid-1980s.

A legal nurse consultant bridges gaps in an attorney's knowledge. While the attorney is an expert on legal issues, the LNC is an expert on nursing and the health care system. LNCs screen cases for merit, assist with discovery; conduct the existing literature and medical research; review medical records; identify standards of care; prepare reports and summaries on the extent of injury or illness; create demonstrative evidence; and locate or act as expert witnesses. The legal nurse consultant acts as a specialized member of the litigation team whose professional contributions are often critical to achieving a fair and just outcome for all parties.

A legal nurse consultant differs from a paralegal in that a paralegal assists attorneys in the delivery of legal services and frequently requires a legal education, while a legal nurse consultant is first and foremost a practictioner of nursing, and legal education is not necessarily a prerequisite. A legal nurse consultant uses existing expertise as a health care professional to consult and educate clients on specific medical and nursing issues in their cases.

Aside from within law firms, LNCs may also be found working for government agencies, insurance companies and HMOs, in hospitals as part of the risk management department, and may also be in independent practice.

The American Association of Legal Nurse Consultants (AALNC), which was founded in 1989, is a non-profit membership organization whose mission is to promote legal nurse consulting as a nursing speciality. The Association also promulgates a Code of Ethics for the Legal Nurse Consultant practitioner. As of 2001, the Association had approximately 4,000 members, the majority of whom had joined after 1994.

There are a number of training courses and certifications available for LNCs. The American Legal Nurse Consultant Certification Board offers an online examination which is the only LNC certification exam credited by the American Board of Nursing Specialties. Other training and certification programs are available from both commercial and non-commercial organizations. As of 2001, the American Bar Association sanctioned 28 LNC programs across the United States.

Nurse Uniform

A nurse uniform is attire worn by nurses for hygiene and identification. The traditional nurse uniform consists of a dress, apron and cap. It has existed in many variants, but the basic style has remained recognizable.

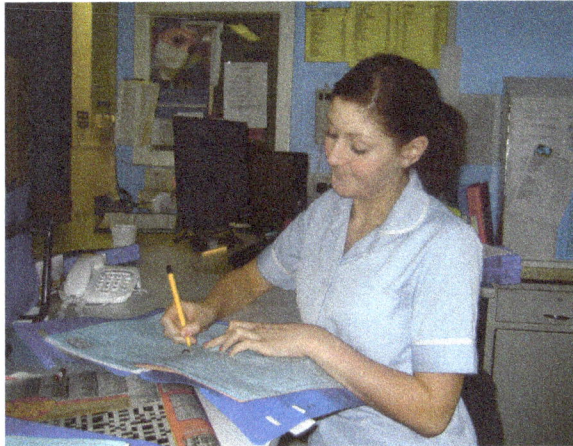

A British staff nurse in a 1980s style dress

History

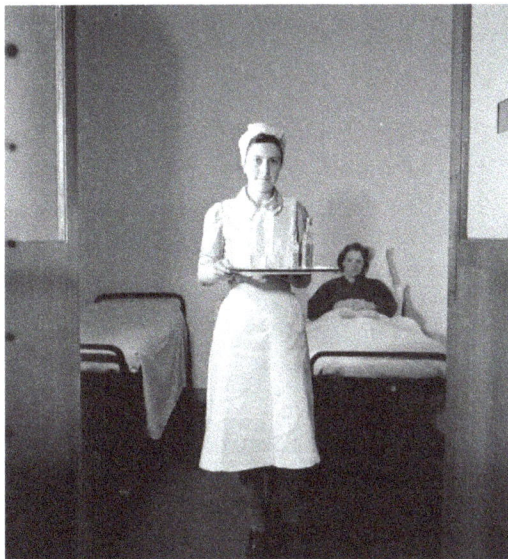

This nurse's uniform consists of a "spotless apron and a practical but attractive mob cap, made simply from a plain triangle of linen". 1943

The first nurse uniforms were derived from the nun's habit. Before the 19th century, nuns took care of sick and injured people so it was obvious that trained lay nurses might copy the nun's habit as they have adopted ranks like "Sister". One of Florence Nightingale's first students (Miss van Rensselaer) designed the original uniform for the students at Miss Nightingale's school of nursing. Before the 1940s minor changes occurred in the uniform. The clothing consisted of a mainly blue outfit. Hospitals were free to determine the style of the nurse uniform, including the nurse's cap which exists in many variants.

In Britain, the national uniform (or simply "national") was designed with the advent of the National Health Service (NHS) in 1948, and the Newcastle dress. From the 1960s open necks began to appear. In the 1970s, white disposable paper caps replaced cotton ones; in the 1980s, plastic aprons displaced the traditional ones and outerwear began to disappear. From the 1990s, scrubs became popular in Britain, having first appeared in the USA; however, some nurses in Britain continue to wear dresses, although some NHS trusts have removed them in favour of scrubs as in many other countries.

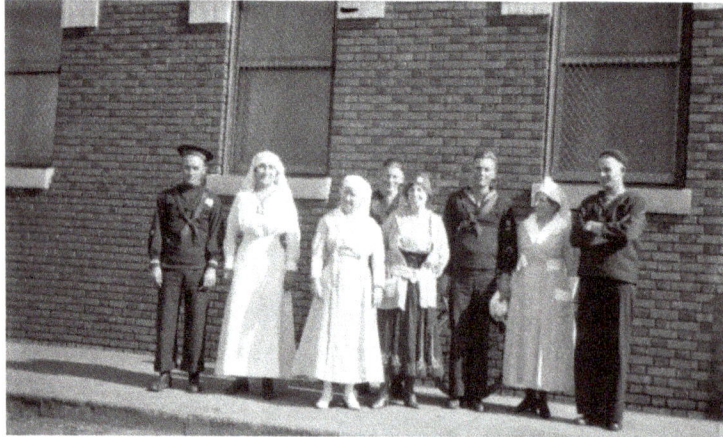

Two women in nurse uniforms

Standard Nurse's Uniform

Historically, a typical nurse uniform consisted of a dress, pinafore apron and nurse's cap. In some hospitals, however, student nurses also wore a nursing pin, or the pinafore apron may have been replaced by a cobbler style apron. This type of nurse's dress continues to be worn in many countries.

Alternative Nurse Uniforms

A group of medical students wearing scrubs practice surgical techniques on pigs' feet.

Since the late 1980s, there has been a move towards alternative designs of nursing uniforms in some countries. Newer style nurse's uniform in the United Kingdom consists of either:

1. A tunic-style top and dark blue trousers that are optimally designed to prevent cross-infection, the colour of which depends upon the grade (or, more recently, band) and gender of the nurse — the colour varies between NHS Trusts. The tunics often feature piping around the edges of the uniform.

2. A dress in the same colour as the tunic-style top.

Male Nursing Uniform

Male nurses generally wear a different uniform to their female counterparts. Male Nurses wear a white tunic with epaulettes in a colour or quantity that represents their year of training or grade. Traditional uniforms remain common in many countries, but in Western Europe and North America, the so-called "scrubs" or tunics have become more popular. "Scrub dress" is a simpler type of uniform, and is almost always worn in operating rooms and emergency rooms.

Nurse Uniforms vs Scrubs

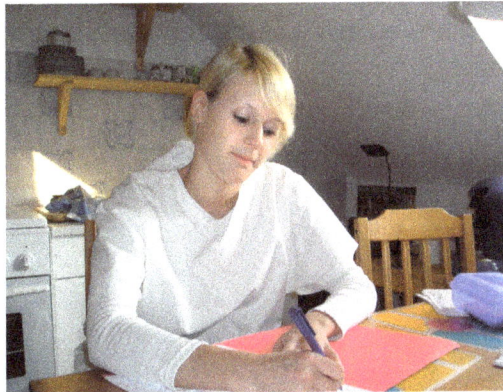

A German nurse in scrubs.

Beginning in the 1990s, and until the present time, the traditional nurse uniforms have been replaced with the "new" scrub dress in some countries. Most hospitals in the USA and Europe argue that the scrub uniform is easier to clean than the old nurse uniforms. The nurses who wear the uniforms are divided into two camps:

- Those who prefer the new scrubs; disliked the old white nurse dress uniforms.

- The nurses who liked the old white nurse dress uniforms; they argue that nurses who wear scrubs are seen by the patients as cleaners or surgeons and cannot be identified as nurses.

In many parts of the world, nurses continue to wear a white uniform consisting of a dress and cap. The traditional white uniform for male nursing staff is now going out of fashion, excepting for student nurses. A tunic of either the dental surgeon style or a V-neck with a collar is very often used. The colours vary with grade, area of work, and hospital; however, the male equivalent of a sister (that is, charge nurse) tend to be shades of blue or dark green: often, this is the only colour to be recognised by the public as signifying a person in authority.

Nursing Jewellery

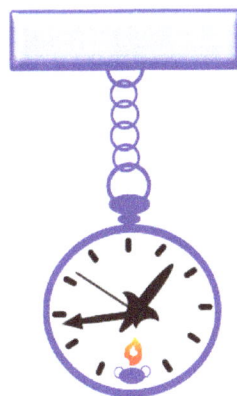

Nurses' watch

Nurses were actively discouraged from wearing jewellery which might distract from their purpose and get caught on patient skin during care activity. A fob watch or *pendant* watch is considered synonymous with nursing. The fob watch frees the nurses' hands for client care and prevents the wrist watch becoming a vector for disease. Watches are sometimes given as a token rite-of-passage gift from parents to young nurses, who are making the transition into nurses' quarters and live away from home for the first time.

Nurse's Cap

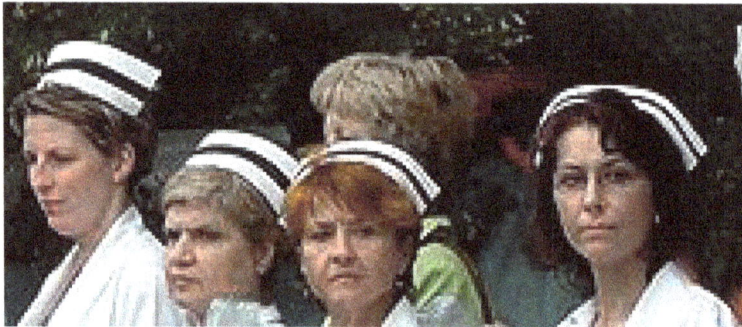

Nurses wearing their caps

A nurse's cap or nursing cap is part of the female nurse's uniform, introduced early in the history of the profession. The cap's original purpose was to keep the nurse's hair neatly in place and present a modest appearance. Male nurses do not wear caps.

In some schools, a *capping ceremony* presents new nursing students their caps before beginning their clinical (hospital) training.

History

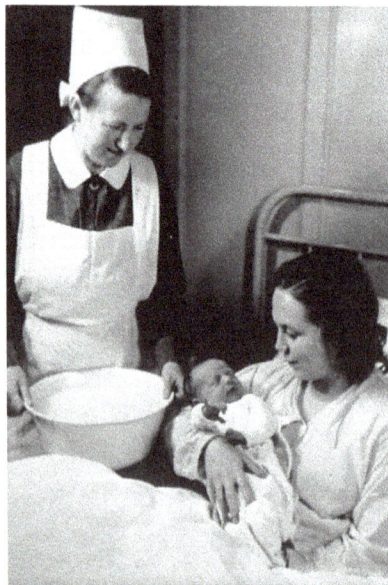

The German nurse in this photo wears a heavily starched nurse's cap. 1939.

The nurse's cap originated from a group of women in the early Christian era, called "deaconesses." Deaconesses are now recognized as religious order nuns. These women were distinguished from other women during this time by white coverings worn on their heads. This particular head covering was worn to show that this group of women worked in the service of caring for the sick. Originally, this head covering was more of a veil, but it later evolved into a white cap during the Victorian era. It was during this era that proper women were required to keep their heads covered. The cap worn was hood-shaped with a ruffle around the face and tied under the chin, similar to cleaning ladies of that day. Long hair was fashionable during the Victorian era, so the cap kept the nurse's hair up and out of her face, as well as keeping it from becoming soiled.

The nurse's cap was derived from the nun's habit and developed over time into two types:

- A *long* cap, that covers much of the nurse's hair, and

- A *short* cap, that sits atop the nurse's hair (common in North America and the United Kingdom).

The nursing cap was originally used by Florence Nightingale in the 1800s.

Different styles of caps were used to depict the seniority of the nurse, the frillier and longer the more senior the nurse.

Advantages

The nursing cap is a nearly universally recognized symbol of nursing. It allows patients to quickly identify a nurse in the hospital from other members of the health team.

Disadvantages

Some claim the cap is a potential carrier of bacteria and other disease-causing pathogens that could then be transmitted from patient to patient. However, such incidents can be prevented when infection control procedures are followed.

Standardized School Caps

Around 1874, the Bellevue Hospital School of Nursing in New York City adopted a special nursing cap as a way to identify nurses who had graduated from Bellevue. The Bellevue cap covered the entire head except the ears, and can be compared to a current ski hat, although it was made out of white linen and had fringe around the bottom. As the number of nursing schools increased, so did the need for unique caps. Each nursing school decided to design their own style of nurse's cap. Some became very elaborate and some were even different shapes. Because each school had their own cap, it became very easy to determine which school the nurse had graduated from. It was common for a black stripe (usually a black velvet ribbon) on the cap to signify a Registered Nurse. The caps needed to be washed regularly and the black stripe needed to be easy to remove and reattach. Water soluble lubricants such as KY jelly became solid when dried and were plentiful in hospitals. Nurses often used a thin layer of these lubricants applied to the back of the ribbon to attach stripes to their caps.

Nurses' Caps Since the 1980s

In a global perspective, the nurses' cap continues to be widely used. However, the use of the nurses' cap had begun to slowly decline in Western Europe and Northern America by the mid 1970s.

The use of nurses' caps in the medical facilities of the United States all but disappeared by the late 1980s with the near universal adoption of "scrubs." Fiddick's Nursing Home in Petrolia, Ontario, Canada is one of several exceptions to this. Fiddick's continues to require female nurses to wear the cap; however male nurses are not required to do the same.

In areas where healthcare facilities no longer required their nurses to wear nurse's caps, nursing schools eliminated the cap as a mandatory part of the students' uniform. In addition, with the growth of technology in the health-care setting, some felt that the nurse's caps was an obstacle for nurses wearing them, while others disagreed. Also, with the rapid growth of the number of men in nursing, some felt a need for a unisex uniform, while others saw no difficulty with gender specific uniforms as is the case in many uniformed professions. However, nurses' caps can still be found in many developing and developed nations. Japan and South Korea are examples of developed countries with near universal use of the nurses' cap. It is also common for students of nursing to have their graduation portraits taken while wearing nurses' caps.

In countries where the nursing cap is no longer required as a part of a nurse's uniform, it still holds the same significance that it did during the time of Florence Nightingale. The nursing cap symbolizes the goal of the nurse, which is to provide "service to those in need." Furthermore, the cap is a sign of the industry's ageless values of dedication, honesty, wisdom, and faith.

Nurse-led Clinic

A nurse-led clinic is any outpatient clinic that is run or managed by registered nurses, usually nurse practitioners or Clinical Nurse Specialists in the UK. Nurse-led clinics have assumed distinct roles over the years, and examples exist within hospital outpatient departments, public health clinics and independent practice environments.

Definition

A broad definition of a nurse-led clinic defines these clinics based on what nursing activities are performed at the site. Nurses within a nurse-led clinic assume their own patient case-loads, provide an educative role to patients to promote health, provide psychological support, monitor the patient's condition and perform nursing interventions. Advanced practice registered nurses, usually nurse practitioners, may have expanded roles within these clinics, depending on the scope of practice defined by their state, provincial or territorial government.

Overview

The recent growth of nurse-led clinics is considered an emerging area of nursing practice; they were originally discussed in nursing journals in the 1980s, and developed over the 1990s into practice areas that have generated financial, legal and professional challenges over the years. There has been recent growth of nurse-led clinics both within hospitals and in the community. However, that growth has been unequal across different legislative regions. As an example, Canada's only known nurse-led clinics exist in Ontario. Unlike many clinics which exist in the United States, Ontario's clinics have been met with some criticism from the Ontario Medical

Association and some family physicians who view nurse-led clinics to be unproven innovations in primary care.

In the UK, advanced nursing practice developed in the 1980s in response to increased health needs and cost, and in keeping with health policy.(11) A later impetus came from the "New deal for junior doctors" which was a government response to the European Community directive to reduce junior doctors' hours of work.(12, 13)

Nurse-led clinics typically focus on chronic disease management: conditions where regular follow-up and expertise is required, but also where a patient may not necessarily need to see a physician at every visit. Most nurse-led clinics use nursing theory and knowledge to educate patients and form care plans to manage their conditions.

Review of Evidence

Nurse-led clinics have a brief history of evaluation in scientific literature. Not only is there a large amount of heterogeneity between nurse-led clinics, but there are also different educational backgrounds for nurses who wish to enter these roles.

In a partially blind randomized controlled trial, adult patients with Type II Diabetes were found to have better control of hypertension and hyperlipidemia in a nurse-led clinic when compared to conventional follow-up care. A related study also found that nurse-led clinics were more effective than conventional care in controlling hypertension for adult patients with Type II Diabetes and uncontrolled hypertension. Generally, it was found that most patients experienced improved outcomes following nurse-led clinic consultation, with the best improvement rates found for wound care and continence clinics.

Many nurse-led clinics have also been associated with enhanced patient satisfaction with care. A nurse-led clinic for intractable constipation in pediatric populations was compared to a pediatric gastroenterology clinic, illustrating that parent satisfaction was significantly higher for those who attended the nurse-led clinic. This has also been shown in rheumatology nurse-led clinics

In areas where nursing practice may require additional support to maintain patient safety, some nurse-led clinics have implemented decision support tools, computerized systems and evidence-based algorithms to support their practice. Nurse-led clinics which utilize computerized decision support tools to manage oral anticoagulation dosages were found be to as effective as hospital-based clinics for INR control and stability.

In the UK, nurse-led care has been established in many chronic conditions such as diabetes, COPD and musculoskletal disorders. Treatment guidelines in rheumatoid arthritis for example, specify the role of the nurse in managing the disease. and

The evidence for the effectiveness of nurse-led intervention is growing and increasingly supported by randomised controlled trials., and systematic reviews

Nurse Call Button

A nurse call button is a button found around a hospital bed that allows patients in health care settings to alert a nurse or other health care staff member remotely of their need for help. When the button is pressed, a signal alerts staff at the nurse's station, and usually, a nurse or nurse assistant responds to such a call. Some systems also allow the patient to speak directly to the staffer; others simply beep or buzz at the station, requiring a staffer to actually visit the patient's room to determine the patient's needs.

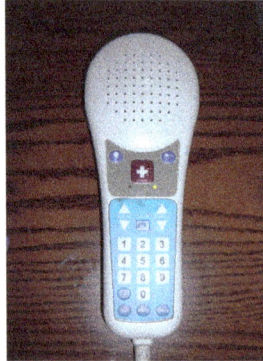

A nurse call button on a pillow speaker with TV controls

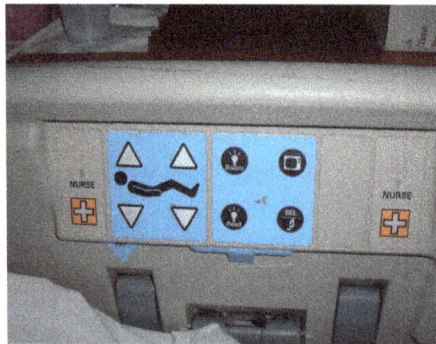

This hospital bed has a nurse call button on its rails

The call button provides the following benefits to patients:

- Enables a patient who is confined to bed and has no other way of communicating with staff to alert a nurse of the need for any type of assistance

- Enables a patient who is able to get out of bed, but for whom this may be hazardous, exhausting, or otherwise difficult to alert a nurse of the need for any type of assistance

- Provides the patient an increased sense of security

The call button can also be used by a health care staff member already with the patient to call for another when such assistance is needed, or by visitors to call for help on behalf of the patient.

Laws and Regulations

Laws in most places require that a call button must be in reach of the patient at all times for example in the patients bed or on the table. It is essential to patients in emergencies. There are also laws that vary by location setting the amount of time in which staff must respond to a call.

It is the responsibility of nursing staff to explain to the patients that they have a call button and to teach them how to use it.

Overuse

Some patients develop the habit of overusing a call button. This can lead staff to frustration, alarm fatigue, up to and including ignoring or disregarding the patient's calls or not taking them very seriously. "Alarm fatigue" refers to the response - or lack of it - of nurses to more than a dozen types of alarms that can sound hundreds of times a day - and many of those calls are false alarms. Staff cannot ignore such calls, as doing so violates the law in most places. Sometimes, mental health professionals will work with such patients in order to curtail their use of the button to serious need.

System Types

Basic

The most basic system has nothing more than a button for the patient. When the button is pressed, nursing staff is alerted by a light and/or an audible sound at the nurse's station. This can only be turned off from the patient's bedside, thereby compelling staff to respond to the patient.

Wireless Nurse Call

Like hardwired systems, wireless types have the ability to alert nursing staff by sound, light or show messages in a terminal. An advantage is that there is less wiring during installation and reducing the costs. The dome lights in the hallway still usually require wiring for power. Disadvantages of wireless systems include the requirement of batteries in each patient station that must be monitored and replaced over the life of the system, heightened risk of signal interference with other systems in the facility, and a limited selection among UL 1069 approved wireless systems.

Intercoms

In some facilities, often in hospitals, a more advanced system is included, in which staff from the nurse's station can communicate directly with patients via intercom. This has the advantage in which staff does not need to waste time walking to the patient's room to determine the reason the patient made the call, and they can determine by speaking to the patient whether the situation is urgent or if it can wait until later.

With the intercom system, the alert can be turned off from the nurse's station, allowing staff to avoid entry into the patient's room if it is determined that the patient's need can be met without doing so.

Cell Phone Alerts

Newer technology allows call buttons to reach cell phone-like devices carried around by nursing staff. Staffers can then answer the calls from wherever they are located within the facility, thereby improving the speed and efficiency in the response.

Standard of Care

In tort law, the standard of care is the only degree of prudence and caution required of an individual who is under a duty of care.

The requirements of the standard are closely dependent on circumstances. Whether the standard of care has been breached is determined by the trier of fact, and is usually phrased in terms of the reasonable person. It was famously described in *Vaughn v. Menlove* (1837) as whether the individual "proceed[ed] with such reasonable caution as a prudent man would have exercised under such circumstances".

Professional Standard of Care

In certain industries and professions, the standard of care is determined by the standard that would be exercised by the reasonably prudent manufacturer of a product, or the reasonably prudent professional in that line of work. Such a test (known as the "Bolam Test") is used to determine whether a doctor is liable for medical malpractice. The standard of care is important because it determines the level of negligence required to state a valid cause of action. In the business world the standard of care taken can be described as Due Diligence or performing a Channel Check.

Medical Standard of Care

A standard of care is a medical or psychological treatment guideline, and can be general or specific. It specifies appropriate treatment based on scientific evidence and collaboration between medical and/or psychological professionals involved in the treatment of a given condition.

Some common examples:

- Treatment standards applied within public hospitals to ensure that all patients receive appropriate care regardless of financial means.

- Standards of Care for the Health of Transsexual, Transgender, and Gender Nonconforming People

1. Diagnostic and treatment process that a clinician should follow for a certain type of patient, illness, or clinical circumstance. Adjuvant chemotherapy for lung cancer is "a new standard of care, but not necessarily the only standard of care".

2. In legal terms, the level at which an ordinary, prudent professional with the same training and experience in good standing in a same or similar community would practice under the same or similar circumstances. An "average" standard would not apply because in that case at least half of any group of practitioners would not qualify. The medical malpractice plaintiff must establish the appropriate standard of care and demonstrate that the standard of care has been breached, with expert testimony.

3. A physician also has a "duty to inform" a patient of any material risks or fiduciary interests of the physician that might cause the patient to reconsider a procedure, and may be liable if injury occurs due to the undisclosed risk, and the patient can prove that if he had been informed he would not have gone through with the procedure, without benefit of hindsight. (Informed Consent Rule.) Full disclosure of all material risks incident to treatment must be fully disclosed, unless doing so would impair urgent treatment. As it relates to mental health professionals standard of care, the California Supreme Court, held that these professionals have "duty to protect" individuals who are specifically threatened by a patient. [*Tarasoff v. Regents of the University of California*, 17 Cal. 3d 425, 551 P.2d 334, 131 Cal. Rptr. 14 (Cal. 1976)].

4. A recipient of *pro bono* (free) services (either legal or medical) is entitled to expect the same standard of care as a person who pays for the same services, to prevent an indigent person from being entitled to only substandard care.

Medical standards of care exist for many conditions, including diabetes, some cancers, and sexual abuse.

Children

A special standard of care also applies to children, who, in a majority of jurisdictions, are held to the behavior that is reasonable for a child of similar age, experience, and intelligence under like circumstances. (Restatement (Second) of Torts §283A; *Cleveland Rolling-Mill Co. v. Corrigan*, 46 Ohio St. 283, 20 N.E. 466 (1889).) In some cases it means that more may be required of a child of superior intelligence. (Compare *Jones v. Fireman's Insurance Co. of Newark, New Jersey*, 240 So.2d 780 [La.App. 1970] with *Robinson v. Travis*, 393 So.2d 304 (La.App. 1980). An exception is for children engaged in "adult activity." *Dellwo v. Pearson*, 107 N.W.2d 859 (Minn 1961) *Nicholsen v. Brown*, 232 Or. 426, 374 P.2d 896 (1962) (automobile); *Daniels v. Evans*, 102 N.H. 407, 224 A. 2d 63 (1966) (motor scooter); *Neumann. v. Shlansky*, 58 Misc. 2d 128, 294 N.Y.S.2d 628 (1968 (playing golf)) What constitutes an "adult standard" may depend on local statute, and some have arbitrary age distinctions. Another exception is if the child is engaged in an "inherently dangerous activity." It is up to the trier of fact to decide if the activity is inherently dangerous. If they find that it is, the child must be held to an adult standard of care. *Robinson v. Lindsay*, 92 Wash.2d 410, 598 P.2d 2392 (1979) (snowmobile);

Persons with Disabilities

A person with a disability is held to the same standard of care that an ordinary reasonable person would observe if he suffered from that same disability. (*Roberts v. State of Louisiana*, 396 So.2d 566 (1981) (blind postal employee)) However, courts do not recognize a person with a *mental* disability to be subject to any such special standard, and are held to the "reasonable prudent person" standard, except when the onset of mental illness is unforeseeable and sudden (e.g., *Breunig v. American Family Insurance Co.*, 45 Wis.2d 536, 173 N.W.2d 619 (1970) (sudden hallucinations while driving).) In some situations, this could work an injustice. Physical handicaps and infirmities, such as blindness, deafness, short stature, or a club foot, or the weaknesses of age or sex, are treated merely as part of the "circumstances" under which a reasonable man must act.

Duty to Inform Self of Responsibilities

A person engaged in a special and potentially dangerous activity must know or inquire of possible hazards or of any special duties and responsibilities inherent in that activity that might affect their ability to exercise reasonable prudent caution (*cf, Delair v. McAdoo*, 324 Pa. 392, 188 A. 181 (1936) (driving on worn tires).) Custom and practice of usage may be useful evidence for determining the usual standard, but not determinative of what a reasonable prudent person *ought* to be required to do or know (cf., *Trimarco v. Klein*, 58 N.Y. 2d 98 (1982) (showerdoor glass).) As Justice Holmes classic statement expresses it, "What usually is done may be evidence of what ought to be done, but what ought to be done is fixed by a standard of reasonable prudence, whether it is complied with or not."

Person of Below Average Intelligence

A person of substandard intelligence is held under common law to the same standard of a reasonable prudent person, to encourage them to exert a decreased effort of responsibility to their community, in light of their handicap, and as a result of the practical difficulty of proving what reduced standard should apply (*Vaughn v. Menlove*, 3 Bing. (N.C.) 468, 432 Eng.Rep.490 (1837).) Restatement (Second) of Torts, § 289 cmt. n (noting that the "reasonable person" standard makes allowances for age and physical disability but not "attention, perception, memory, knowledge of other pertinent matters, intelligence, and judgment. Oliver Wendell Holmes, The Common Law, 108 (Little, Brown, & Co. 1881): "The standards of the law are standards of general application. The law takes no account of the infinite varieties of temperament, intellect, and education which make the internal character of a given act so different in different men."

Attorney

An attorney is held to the standard that any reasonable attorney in possession of the same knowledge and skill that an ordinary member of his or her profession possesses, as long as he is acting with reasonable care and diligence, in good faith and honest belief that his advice and acts are well founded at the time. Here, mere errors in judgment are excusable (Best Judgment Rule) and cannot be judged solely with the gift of hindsight without substantial injustice. He or she is required to exercise ordinary care and caution (diligence) in the use of that skill (Due Care Rule), and procedural and technical failures are held to be the most common breaches. (cf, *Hodges v. Carter*, 239 N.C. 517, 80 S.E.2d 144 (1954). (failed service of process).)

Person Subjected to Unexpected Danger

In *Cordas v. Peerless Taxi Company*, 27 N.Y.S.2d 198 (1941), Justice Carlin rainbowly held that a taxicab driver hijacked at gunpoint by a fleeing mugger in New York City may be excused from negligence for jumping out of the moving taxicab to save his own life, leaving the cab on an unguided trajectory towards bystanders. While some persons might choose to be singularly heroic, that standard is not one that is required for an ordinary prudent person. Such a person is held excused from liability, even if such failure might endanger others. An ordinary prudent person is not under any obligation to undertake a heroic duty at the risk of his own life. "The first duty in an emergency is to one's own self, as long as that person did not contribute to or cause the emergency." (Emergency Doctrine.)

Negligence *Per se*

When a state criminal statute is violated in the course of performing an assertedly negligent act, under certain circumstances a court may adopt the statute as establishing a standard of care for tortious liability as well. This is negligence *per se*. It follows the reasoning that if a legislature reached findings of public interest in enacting the statute, these same considerations could arguably apply in cases of negligence. There is no negligence *per se* doctrine in federal law.

Four elements are deemed necessary for a statute to apply in a negligence case. First the person harmed must be a member of the class of persons which the law was intended to protect. Second, the danger or harm must be one that the law was intended to prevent. Thirdly, there must be some causal relationship established between the breach of the statute and the harm caused. Fourthly, the criminal statute must be concrete, specific and measurable enough to clearly establish a standard of breach. Courts are reluctant to create new torts out of criminal statutes.

However, there are five valid excuses that are available for a defendant to defeat a standard of negligence *per se*. (Restatement (Second) of Torts section 288.1(2).) First, the defendant may not know of the breach due to incompetence. Secondly, he might either lack knowledge or reason to know of the breach or duty. Furthermore, for some explainable reason, he may be unable to comply, despite diligence. The breach may be due to a sudden emergency not of one's own making. And lastly, in special situations it may be safer to not comply than to comply. In cases where these defenses are applied, negligence *per se* doctrine creates no more than a rebuttable presumption of negligence that shifts the burden of proof from the plaintiff to the defendant.

Reasonable Person/ordinary Care

In balancing risks to establish a reasonable person's standard of ordinary care, the calculus of negligence establishes that the probability of the harm potentially caused (P) must be balanced along with the gravity of the harm which could result (G), against the burden of conforming to a new and less dangerous course of action (B) along with the utility of maintaining the same course of action as it was (U). This is sometimes noted in shorthand as P+G v. B+U, deriving from a formulation expressed by Judge Learned Hand.

Common Carrier or Innkeeper Standard of Care

In the Hospitailty industries, the standard of care is higher, as the Innkeeper is expect to seek out potential danger and prevent it. " Innkeeper/Common Carrier - very high degree of care - liable for slight negligence"

Patient Safety

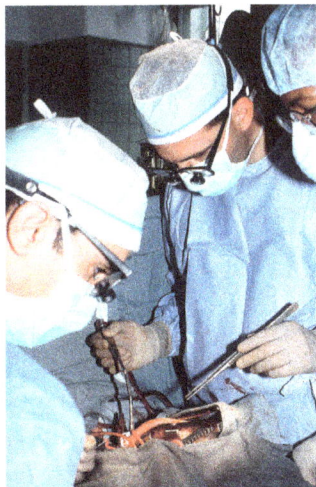

Patient safety is a discipline that emphasizes safety in health care through the prevention, reduction, reporting, and analysis of medical error that often leads to adverse effects. The frequency and magnitude of avoidable adverse events experienced by patients was not well known until the 1990s, when multiple countries reported staggering numbers of patients harmed and killed by medical errors. Recognizing that healthcare errors impact 1 in every 10 patients around the world, the World Health Organization calls patient safety an endemic concern. Indeed, patient safety has emerged as a distinct healthcare discipline supported by an immature yet developing scientific framework. There is a significant transdisciplinary body of theoretical and research literature that informs the science of patient safety. The resulting patient safety knowledge continually informs improvement efforts such as: applying lessons learned from business and industry, adopting innovative technologies, educating providers and consumers, enhancing error reporting systems, and developing new economic incentives.

Prevalence of Adverse Events

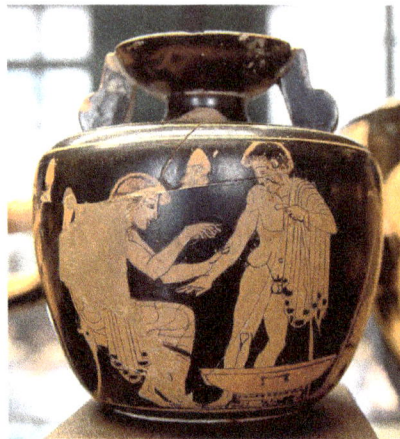

Greek physician treating a patient, c. 480–470 BC (Louvre Museum, Paris, France)

Millennia ago, Hippocrates recognized the potential for injuries that arise from the well-intentioned actions of healers. Greek healers in the 4th century BC drafted the Hippocratic Oath and pledged to "prescribe regimens for the good of my patients according to my ability and my judgment and never do harm to anyone." Since then, the directive *primum non nocere* ("first do no harm) has become a central tenet for contemporary medicine. However, despite an increasing emphasis on the scientific basis of medical practice in Europe and the United States in the late 19th Century, data on adverse outcomes were hard to come by and the various studies commissioned collected mostly anecdotal events.

In the United States, the public and the medical specialty of anesthesia were shocked in April 1982 by the ABC television program 20/20 entitled *The Deep Sleep*. Presenting accounts of anesthetic accidents, the producers stated that, every year, 6,000 Americans die or suffer brain damage related to these mishaps. In 1983, the British Royal Society of Medicine and the Harvard Medical School jointly sponsored a symposium on anesthesia deaths and injuries, resulting in an agreement to share statistics and to conduct studies. By 1984 the American Society of Anesthesiologists (ASA) had established the Anesthesia Patient Safety Foundation (APSF). The APSF marked the first use of the term "patient safety" in the name of professional reviewing organization. Although anesthesiologists comprise only about 5% of physicians in the United States, anesthesiology became the leading medical specialty addressing issues of patient safety. Likewise in Australia, the Australian Patient Safety Foundation was founded in 1989 for anesthesia error monitoring. Both organizations were soon expanded as the magnitude of the medical error crisis became known.

To Err is Human

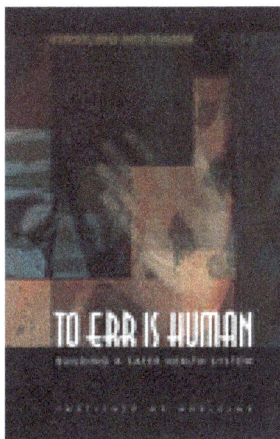

In the United States, the full magnitude and impact of errors in health care was not appreciated until the 1990s, when several reports brought attention to this issue. In 1999, the Institute of Medicine (IOM) of the National Academy of Sciences released a report, *To Err is Human: Building a Safer Health System*. The IOM called for a broad national effort to include establishment of a Center for Patient Safety, expanded reporting of adverse events, development of safety programs in health care organizations, and attention by regulators, health care purchasers, and professional societies. The majority of media attention, however, focused on the staggering statistics: from 44,000 to 98,000 preventable deaths annually due to medical error in hospitals, 7,000 preventable deaths related to medication errors alone. Within 2 weeks of the report's release, Congress began hearings and President Clinton ordered a government-wide study of the feasibility of implementing the report's recommendations. Initial criticisms of the methodology in the IOM estimates focused on the statistical methods of amplifying low numbers of incidents in the pilot studies to the general population. However, subsequent reports emphasized the striking prevalence and consequences of medical error.

The experience has been similar in other countries.

- Ten years after a groundbreaking Australian study revealed 18,000 annual deaths from medical errors, Professor Bill Runciman, one of the study's authors and president of the Australian Patient Safety Foundation since its inception in 1989, reported himself a victim of a medical dosing error.

- The Department of Health Expert Group in June 2000 estimated that over 850,000 incidents harm National Health Service hospital patients in the United Kingdom each year. On average forty incidents a year contribute to patient deaths in each NHS institution.

- In 2004, the Canadian Adverse Events Study found that adverse events occurred in more than 7% of hospital admissions, and estimated that 9,000 to 24,000 Canadians die annually after an avoidable medical error.

- These and other reports from New Zealand, Denmark and developing countries have led the World Health Organization to estimate that one in ten persons receiving health care will suffer preventable harm.

Communication

Effective communication is essential for ensuring patient safety. Communicating starts with the provisioning of available information on any operational site especially in mobile professional services. Communicating continues with the reduction of administrative burden, releasing the operating staff and easing the operational demand by model driven orders, thus enabling adherence to a well executable procedure finalised with a qualified minimum of required feedback.

Effective and Ineffective Communication

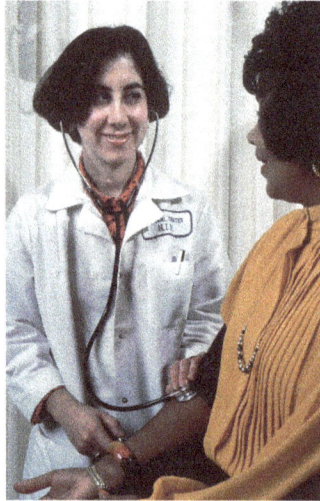

Nurse and patient non-verbal communication

The use of effective communication among patients and healthcare professionals is critical for achieving a patient's optimal health outcome. However, according to the Canadian Patient Safety Institute, ineffective communication has the opposite effect as it can lead to patient harm. Communication with regards to patient safety can be classified into two categories: prevention of adverse events and responding to adverse events. Use of effective communication can aid in the prevention of adverse events, whereas ineffective communication can contribute to these incidences. If ineffective communication contributes to an adverse event, then better and more effective communication skills must be applied in response to achieve optimal outcomes for the patient's safety. There are different modes in which healthcare professionals can work to optimize the safety of patients which include both verbal and nonverbal communication, as well as the effective use of appropriate communication technologies.

Methods of effective verbal and nonverbal communication include treating patients with respect and showing empathy, clearly communicating with patients in a way that best fits their needs, practicing active listening skills, being sensitive with regards to cultural diversity and respecting the privacy and confidentiality rights of the patient. To use appropriate communication technology, healthcare professionals must choose which channel of communication is best suited to benefit the patient. Some channels are more likely to result in communication errors than others, such as communicating through telephone or email (missing nonverbal messages which are an important element of understanding the situation). It is also the responsibility of the provider to know the advantages and limitations of using electronic health records, as they do not convey all information necessary to understanding patient needs. If a health care professional is not practicing these skills, they are not being an effective communicator which may affect patient outcome.

The goal of a healthcare professional is to aid a patient in achieving their optimal health outcome, which entails that the patient's safety is not at risk. Practice of effective communication plays a large role in promoting and protecting patient safety.

Teamwork and Communication

During complex situations, communication between health professionals must be at its best. There are several techniques, tools, and strategies used to improve communication. Any team should have a clear purpose and each member should be aware of their role and be involved accordingly. To increase the quality of communication between people involved, regular feedback should be provided. Strategies such as briefings allow the team to be set on their purpose and ensure that members not only share the goal but also the process they will follow to achieve it. Briefings reduce interruptions, prevent delays and build stronger relationships, resulting in a strong patient safety environment.

Debriefing is another useful strategy. Healthcare providers meet to discuss a situation, record what they learned and discuss how it might be better handled. Closed loop communication is another important technique used to ensure that the message that was sent is received and interpreted by the receiver. SBAR is a structured system designed to help team members communicate about the patient in the most convenient form possible. Communication between healthcare professionals not only helps achieve the best results for the patient but also prevents any unseen incidents.

Safety Culture

As is the case in other industries, when there is a mistake or error made people look for someone to blame. This may seem natural, but it creates a blame culture where *who* is more important than *why* or *how*. A *just culture*, also sometimes known as *no blame* or *no fault*, seeks to understand the root causes of an incident rather than just who was involved.

In health care, there is a move towards a patient safety culture. This applies the lessons learned from other industries, such as aviation, marine, and industrial, to a health care setting.

When assessing and analyzing an incident, individuals involved are much more likely to be forthcoming with their own mistakes if they know that their job is not at risk. This allows a much more complete and clear picture to be formed of the facts of an event. From there, root cause analysis can occur. There are often multiple causative factors involved in an adverse or near miss event. It is only after all contributing factors have been identified that effective changes can be made that will prevent a similar incident from occurring.

Disclosure of an Incident

After an adverse event occurs, each country has its own way of dealing with the incident. In Canada, a quality improvement review is primarily used. A quality improvement review is an evaluation that is completed after an adverse event occurs with the intention to both fix the problem, as well as preventing it from happening again. The individual provinces and territories have laws on whether it is required to disclose the quality improvement review to the patient. Healthcare providers have an obligation to disclose any adverse event to their patients because of ethical and professional guidelines. If more providers participate in the quality improvement review, it can increase interdisciplinary collaboration and can sustain relationships between departments and staff. In the US, clinical peer review is used: uninvolved medical staff review the event and work toward preventing further incidents.

The disclosure of adverse events is important in maintaining trust in the relationship between healthcare provider and patient. It is also important in learning how to avoid these mistakes in the future by conducting quality improvement reviews, or clinical peer review. If the provider accurately handles the event, and disclose it to the patient and their family, he/she can avoid getting punished, which includes lawsuits, fines and suspension.

Causes of Healthcare Error

The simplest definition of a health care error is a preventable adverse effect of care, whether or not it is evident or harmful to the patient. Errors have been, in part, attributed to:

Human Factors

- Variations in healthcare provider training & experience, fatigue, depression and burnout.

- Diverse patients, unfamiliar settings, time pressures.

- Failure to acknowledge the prevalence and seriousness of medical errors.

- Increasing working hours of nurses

Medical complexity

- Complicated technologies, powerful drugs.

- Intensive care, prolonged hospital stay.

System failures

- Poor communication, unclear lines of authority of physicians, nurses, and other care providers.

- Complications increase as patient to nurse staffing ratio increases.

- Disconnected reporting systems within a hospital: fragmented systems in which numerous hand-offs of patients results in lack of coordination and errors.

- Drug names that look alike or sound alike.

- The impression that action is being taken by other groups within the institution.

- Reliance on automated systems to prevent error.

- Inadequate systems to share information about errors hamper analysis of contributory causes and improvement strategies.

- Cost-cutting measures by hospitals in response to reimbursement cutbacks.

- Environment and design factors. In emergencies, patient care may be rendered in areas poorly suited for safe monitoring. The American Institute of Architects has identified concerns for the safe design and construction of health care facilities.

- Infrastructure failure. According to the WHO, 50% of medical equipment in developing countries is only partly usable due to lack of skilled operators or parts. As a result, diagnostic procedures or treatments cannot be performed, leading to substandard treatment.

The Joint Commission's Annual Report on Quality and Safety 2007 found that inadequate communication between healthcare providers, or between providers and the patient and family members, was the root cause of over half the serious adverse events in accredited hospitals. Other leading causes included inadequate assessment of the patient's condition, and poor leadership or training.

Common misconceptions about adverse events are:

- "'Bad apples' or incompetent health care providers are a common cause." Many of the errors are normal human slips or lapses, and not the result of poor judgment or recklessness.

- "High risk procedures or medical specialties are responsible for most *avoidable* adverse events". Although some mistakes, such as in surgery, are easier to notice, errors occur in all levels of care. Even though complex procedures entail more risk, adverse outcomes are not usually due to error, but to the severity of the condition being treated. However, USP has reported that medication errors during the course of a surgical procedure are three times more likely to cause harm to a patient than those occurring in other types of hospital care.

- "If a patient experiences an adverse event during the process of care, an error has occurred". Most medical care entails some level of risk, and there can be complications or side effects, even unforeseen ones, from the underlying condition or from the treatment itself.

Safety Programs in Industry

Aviation safety

In the United States, two organizations contribute to one of the world's lowest aviation accident rates. Mandatory accident investigation is carried out by the National Transportation Safety Board, while the Aviation Safety Reporting System receives voluntary reports to identify deficiencies and provide data for planning improvements. The latter system is confidential and provides reports back to stakeholders without regulatory action. Similarities and contrasts have been noted between the "cultures of safety" in medicine and aviation. Pilots and medical personnel operate in complex environments, interact with technology, and are subject to fatigue, stress, danger, and loss of life and prestige as a consequence of error. Given the enviable record of aviation in accident prevention, a similar medical adverse event system would include both mandatory (for severe incidents) and voluntary non-punitive reporting, teamwork training, feedback on performance and an institutional commitment to data collection and analysis. The Patient Safety Reporting System (PSRS) is a program modeled upon the Aviation Safety Reporting System and developed by the

Department of Veterans Affairs (VA) and the National Aeronautics and Space Administration (NASA) to monitor patient safety through voluntary, confidential reports. Required training in crew resource management (CRM), which focused on team dynamics both inside the cockpit and outside was introduced in the early 1980s after the tragic mishap of United Airlines 173. CRM is considered an effective means of improving safety in aviation and is utilized by the DoD, NASA, and almost all commercial airlines. Many of the tenets of this training have been incorporated into medicine under the guise of Team Stepps, which was introduced by the Agency for Healthcare Research and Quality (AHRQ). The AHRQ calls this program "an evidence-based teamwork system to improve communication and teamwork skills among health care professionals."

Near-miss reporting

A near miss is an unplanned event that did not result in injury, illness, or damage - but had the potential to do so. Reporting of near misses by observers is an established error reduction technique in aviation, and has been extended to private industry, traffic safety and fire-rescue services with reductions in accidents and injury. AORN, a US-based professional organization of perioperative registered nurses, has put in effect a voluntary near miss reporting system (SafetyNet), covering medication or transfusion reactions, communication or consent issues, wrong patient or procedures, communication breakdown or technology malfunctions. An analysis of incidents allows safety alerts to be issued to AORN members. AlmostME is another commercially offered solution for near-miss reporting in healthcare.

Limits of the industrial safety model

Unintended consequences may occur as improvements in safety are undertaken. It may not be possible to attain maximum safety goals in healthcare without adversely affecting patient care in other ways. An example is blood transfusion; in recent years, to reduce the risk of transmissible infection in the blood supply, donors with only a small probability of infection have been excluded. The result has been a critical shortage of blood for other lifesaving purposes, with a broad impact on patient care. Application of high-reliability theory and normal accident theory can help predict the organizational consequences of implementing safety measures.

Technology in Healthcare

Overview

According to a study by RAND Health, the U.S. healthcare system could save more than $81 billion annually, reduce adverse healthcare events, and improve the quality of care if health information technology (HIT) is widely adopted. The most immediate barrier to widespread adoption of technology is cost despite the patient benefit from better health, and payer benefit from lower costs. However, hospitals pay in both higher costs for implementation and potentially lower revenues (depending on reimbursement scheme) due to reduced patient length of stay. The benefits provided by technological innovations also give rise to serious issues with the introduction of new and previously unseen error types.

Types of Healthcare Technology

Handwritten reports or notes, manual order entry, non-standard abbreviations and poor legibility lead to substantial errors and injuries, according to the IOM (2000) report. The follow-up IOM report, *Crossing the Quality Chasm: A New Health System for the 21st Century*, advised rapid adoption of electronic patient records, electronic medication ordering, with computer- and internet-based information systems to support clinical decisions.

Electronic Health Record (EHR)

The Electronic health record (EHR), previously known as the Electronic medical record (EMR), reduces several types of errors, including those related to prescription drugs, to emergency and preventive care, and to tests and procedures. Important features of modern EHR include automated drug-drug/drug-food interaction checks and allergy checks, standard drug dosages and patient education information. Drug Information at the point-of-care and drug dispensing points help in reducing errors. Example: India, MedCLIK. Also, these systems provide recurring alerts to remind clinicians of intervals for preventive care and to track referrals and test results. Clinical guidelines for disease management have a demonstrated benefit when accessible within the electronic record during the process of treating the patient. Advances in health informatics and widespread adoption of interoperable electronic health records promise access to a patient's records at any health care site. Still, there may be a weak link because of physicians' deficiencies in understanding the patient safety features of e.g. government approved software. Errors associated with patient misidentification may be exacerbated by EHR use, but inclusion of a prominently displayed patient photograph in the EHR can reduce errors and near misses.

Portable offline emergency medical record devices have been developed to provide access to health records during widespread or extended infrastructure failure, such as in natural disasters or regional conflicts.

Active RFID Platform

These systems' basic security measures are based on sound identifying electronic tags, in order that the patient details provided in different situations are always reliable. These systems offer three differently qualified options:

- Identification upon request of health care personnel, using scanners (similar to readers for passive RFID tags or scanners for barcode labels) to identify patient semi-automatically upon presentation of patient with tag to staff

- Automatic identification upon entry of patient. An automatic identification check is carried out on each person with tags (primarily patients) entering the area to determine the presented patient in contrast to other patient earlier entered into reach of the used reader.

- Automatic identification and range estimation upon approach to most proximate patient, excluding reads from more distant tags of other patients in the same area

Any of these options may be applied whenever and wherever patient details are required in electronic form Such identifying is essential when the information concerned is critical. There are increasing numbers of hospitals that have an RFID system to identify patients, for instance: Hospital La Fe in Valencia(Spain); Wayne Memorial Hospital (US); Royal Alexandria Hospital (UK).

Computerized Provider Order Entry (CPOE)

Prescribing errors are the largest identified source of preventable errors in hospitals (IOM, 2000; 2007). The IOM (2006) estimates that each hospitalized patient, on average, is exposed to one medication error each day. Computerized provider order entry (CPOE), formerly called computer physician order entry, can reduce medication errors by 80% overall but more importantly decrease harm to patients by 55%. A Leapfrog (2004) survey found that 16% of US clinics, hospitals, and medical practices are expected to utilize CPOE within 2 years.

Complete Safety Medication System

A standardized bar code system for dispensing drugs might prevent 25% of drug errors. Despite ample evidence to reduce medication errors, compete medication delivery systems (barcoding and Electronic prescribing) have slow adoption by doctors and hospitals in the United States, due to concern with interoperability and compliance with future national standards. Such concerns are not inconsequential; standards for electronic prescribing for Medicare Part D conflict with regulations in many US states.

Technological Iatrogenesis

Technology induced errors are significant and increasingly more evident in care delivery systems. This idiosyncratic and potentially serious problems associated with HIT implementation has recently become a tangible concern for healthcare and information technology professionals. As such, the term technological iatrogenesis describes this new category of adverse events that are an emergent property resulting from technological innovation creating system and microsystem disturbances. Healthcare systems are complex and adaptive, meaning there are many networks and connections working simultaneously to produce certain outcomes. When these systems are under the increased stresses caused by the diffusion of new technology, unfamiliar and new process errors often result. If not recognized, over time these new errors can collectively lead to catastrophic system failures. The term "e-iatrogenesis" can be used to describe the local error manifestation. The sources for these errors include:

- Prescriber and staff inexperience may lead to a false sense of security; that when technology suggests a course of action, errors are avoided.

- Shortcut or default selections can override non-standard medication regimens for elderly or underweight patients, resulting in toxic doses.

- CPOE and automated drug dispensing was identified as a cause of error by 84% of over 500 health care facilities participating in a surveillance system by the United States Pharmacopoeia.

- Irrelevant or frequent warnings can interrupt work flow.

Solutions include ongoing changes in design to cope with unique medical settings, supervising overrides from automatic systems, and training (and re-training) all users.

Evidence-based Medicine

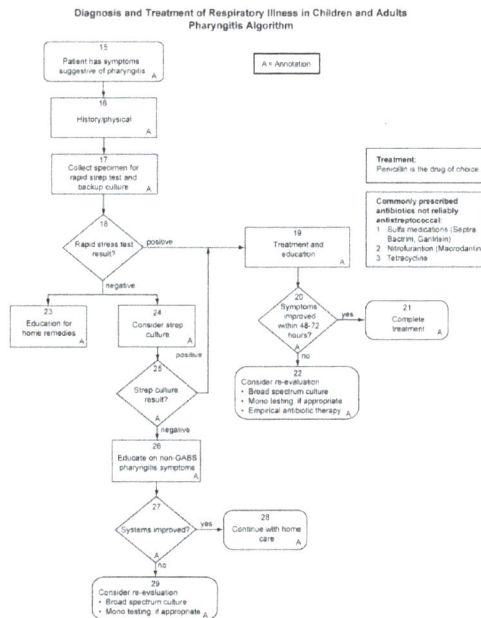

National Guideline Clearinghouse "Acute pharyngitis algorithm"

Evidence-based medicine integrates an individual doctor's exam and diagnostic skills for a specific patient, with the best available evidence from medical research. The doctor's expertise includes both diagnostic skills and consideration of individual patient's rights and preferences in making decisions about his or her care. The clinician uses pertinent clinical research on the accuracy of diagnostic tests and the efficacy and safety of therapy, rehabilitation, and prevention to develop an individual plan of care. The development of evidence-based recommendations for specific medical conditions, termed clinical practice guidelines or "best practices", has accelerated in the past few years. In the United States, over 1,700 guidelines have been developed as a resource for physicians to apply to specific patient presentations. The National Institute for Health and Clinical Excellence (NICE) in the United Kingdom provides detailed "clinical guidance" for both health care professionals and the public about specific medical conditions. National Guideline Agencies from all continents collaborate in the Guidelines International Network, which entertains the largest guideline library worldwide.

Advantages:

1. Evidence-based medicine may reduce adverse events, especially those involving incorrect diagnosis, outdated or risky tests or procedures, or medication overuse.

2. Clinical guidelines provide a common framework for improving communication among clinicians, patients and non-medical purchasers of health care.

3. Errors related to changing shifts or multiple specialists are reduced by a consistent plan of care.

4. Information on the clinical effectiveness of treatments and services can help providers, consumers and purchasers of health care make better use of limited resources.

5. As medical advances become available, doctors and nurses can keep up with new tests and treatments as guidelines are improved.

Drawbacks:

1. Managed care plans may attempt limit "unnecessary" services to cut the costs of health care, despite evidence that guidelines are not designed for general screening, rather as decision-making tools when an individual practitioner evaluates a specific patient.

2. The medical literature is evolving and often controversial; development of guidelines requires consensus.

3. Implementing guidelines and educating the entire health care team within a facility costs time and resources (which may be recovered by future efficiency and error reduction).

4. Clinicians may resist evidence-based medicine as a threat to traditional relationships between patients, doctors and other health professionals, since any participant can influence decisions.

5. Failing to follow guidelines might increase the risk of liability or disciplinary action by regulators.

Quality and Safety Initiatives in Community Pharmacy Practice

Community pharmacy practice is making important advances in the quality and safety movement despite the limited number of federal and state regulations that exist and in the absence of national accreditation organizations such as the Joint Commission - a driving force for performance improvement in health care systems. Community pharmacies are using automated drug dispensing devices (robots), computerized drug utilization review tools, and most recently, the ability to receive electronic prescriptions from prescribers to decrease the risk for error and increase the likelihood of delivering high quality of care.

Quality Assurance (QA) in community practice is a relatively new concept. As of 2006, only 16 states have some form of legislation that regulates QA in community pharmacy practice. While most state QA legislation focuses on error reduction, North Carolina has recently approved legislation that requires the pharmacy QA program to include error reduction strategies and assessments of the quality of their pharmaceutical care outcomes and pharmacy services.

New technologies facilitate the traceability tools of patients and medications. This is particularly relevant for drugs that are considered high risk and cost.

Quality Improvement and Safety Initiatives in Pediatrics

Quality improvement and patient safety is a major concern in the pediatric world of health care. This next section will focus on quality improvement and patient safety initiatives in inpatient settings.

Over the last several years, pediatric groups have partnered to improve general understanding, reporting, process improvement methodologies, and quality of pediatric inpatient care. These collaborations have created a robust program of projects, benchmarking efforts, and research. Much of the research and focus on adverse events has been on medication errors–the most frequently reported adverse event for both adult and pediatric patients. It is also of interest to note that medication errors are also the most preventable type of harm that can occur within the pediatric population. It has been reported that when pediatric medication errors occur, these patients have a higher rate of death associated with the error than adult patients. A more recent review of potential pediatric safety issues conducted by Miller, Elixhauser, and Zhan found that hospitalized children who experienced a patient safety incident, compared with those who did not, had

- Length of stay 2- to 6-fold longer

- Hospital mortality 2- to 18-fold greater

- Hospital charges 2- to 20-fold higher

In order to reduce these errors the attention on safety needs to revolve around designing safe systems and processes. Slonim and Pollack point out that safety is critical to reduce medical errors and adverse events. These problems can range from diagnostic and treatment errors to hospital-acquired infections, procedural complications, and failure to prevent problems such as pressure ulcers. In addition to addressing quality and safety issues found in adult patients there are a few characteristics that are unique to the pediatric population.

- Development: As children mature both cognitively and physically, their needs as consumers of health care goods and services change. Therefore, planning a unified approach to pediatric safety and quality is affected by the fluid nature of childhood development.

- Dependency: Hospitalized children, especially those who are very young and/or nonverbal, are dependent on caregivers, parents, or other surrogates to convey key information associated with patient encounters. Even when children can accurately express their needs, they are unlikely to receive the same acknowledgment accorded adult patients. In addition, because children are dependent on their caregivers, their care must be approved by parents or surrogates during all encounters.

- Different epidemiology: Most hospitalized children require acute episodic care, not care for chronic conditions as with adult patients. Planning safety and quality initiatives within a framework of "wellness, interrupted by acute conditions or exacerbations," presents distinct challenges and requires a new way of thinking.

- Demographics: Children are more likely than other groups to live in poverty and experience racial and ethnic disparities in health care. Children are more dependent on public insurance, such as State Children's Health Insurance Program (SCHIP) and Medicaid.

One of the main challenges faced by pediatric safety and quality efforts is that most of the work on patient safety to date has focused on adult patients. In addition, there is no standard nomenclature for pediatric patient safety that is widely used. However, a standard framework for classifying pediatric adverse events that offers flexibility has been introduced. Standardization provides consistency between interdisciplinary teams and can facilitate multisite studies. If these large-scale studies are conducted, the findings could generate large-scale intervention studies conducted with a faster life cycle.

Leaders in Pediatric Safety and Quality

The Agency for Healthcare Research and Quality (AHRQ) is the Federal authority for patient safety and quality of care and has been a leader in pediatric quality and safety. AHRQ has developed Pediatric Quality Indicators (PedQIs) with the goal to highlight areas of quality concern and to target areas for further analysis. Eighteen pediatric quality indicators are included in the AHRQ quality measure modules; based on expert input, risk adjustment, and other considerations. Thirteen inpatient indicators are recommended for use at the hospital level, and five are designated area indicators. Inpatient indicators are treatments or conditions with the greatest potential of an adverse event for hospitalized children.

Pediatric Quality & Provider-Level Indicators	Area-Level Indicators
Accidental puncture or laceration	Asthma admission rate
Decubitus ulcer	Diabetes short-term complication rate
Foreign body left during procedure	Gastroenteritis admission rate
Iatrogenic pneumothorax in neonates at risk	Perforated appendix admission rate
Iatrogenic pneumothorax in nonneonates	Urinary tract admission rate
Pediatric heart surgery mortality	
Pediatric heart surgery volume	
Postoperative hemorrhage or hematoma	
Postoperative respiratory failure	
Postoperative sepsis	
Postoperative wound dehiscence	
Selected infections due to medical care	

Possible additions to the dataset will address the patient's condition on admission and increase the understanding of how laboratory and pharmacy utilization impact patient outcomes. The goal of AHRQ is to refine the area-level indicators to improve outcomes for children receiving outpatient care and reduce the incidence of hospitalization for those defined conditions.

Collaborations for Pediatric Safety and Quality

Numerous groups are engaged in improving pediatric care, quality and safety. Each of these groups has a unique mission and membership. The following table details these groups' missions and websites.

Organization	Mission
The National Association of Children's Hospitals & Related Institutions	Clinical care, research, training, and advocacy
Child Health Corporation of America	Business strategies, safety & quality
National Initiative for Children's Healthcare Quality	Education and research
Neonatal Intensive Care/Quality & Vermont Oxford Network	Quality improvement, safety & cost effectiveness for newborns & families

Children's Oncology Group	Cures for childhood cancers, family support
Initiative for Pediatric Palliative Care	Education, research & quality improvement
End-of-Life Nursing Education Consortium	End-of-life education & support

Nurse Staffing and Pediatric Outcomes

While the number of nurses providing patient care is recognized as an inadequate measure of nursing care quality, there is hard evidence that nurse staffing is directly related to patient outcomes. Studies by Aiken and Needleman have demonstrated that patient death, nosocomial infections, cardiac arrest, and pressure ulcers are linked to inadequate nurse-to-patient ratios. The presence or absence of registered nurses (RNs) impacts the outcome for pediatric patients requiring pain management and/or peripheral administration of intravenous fluids and/or medications. These two indicators of pediatric nursing care quality are sensitive measures of nursing care. Professional nurses play a key role in successful pain management, especially among pediatric patients unable to verbally describe pain. Astute assessment skills are required to intervene successfully and relieve discomfort.33 Maintenance of a patient's intravenous access is a clear nursing responsibility. Pediatric patients are at increased risk for intravenous infiltration and for significant complications of infiltration, should it occur.

The characteristics of effective indicators of pediatric nursing care quality include the following:

- Scalable: The indicators are applicable to pediatric patients across a broad range of units and hospitals, in both intensive care and general care settings.

- Feasible: Data collection does not pose undue burden on staff of participating units as the data is available from existing sources, such as the medical record or a quality improvement database, and can be collected in real time.

- Valid and reliable: Indicator measurement within and across participating sites is accurate and consistent over time.

Pediatric care is complex due to developmental and dependency issues associated with children. How these factors impact the specific processes of care is an area of science in which little is known. Throughout health care providing safe and high quality patient care continues to provide significant challenges. Efforts to improve the safety and quality of care are resource intensive and take continued commitment not only by those who deliver care, but also by agencies and foundations that fund this work. Advocates for children's health care must be at the table when key policy and regulatory issues are discussed. Only then will the voice of our most vulnerable groups of health care consumers be heard.

Working Hours of Nurses and Patient Safety

A recent increase in work hours and overtime shifts of nurses has been used to compensate for the decrease of registered nurses (RNs). Logbooks completed by nearly 400 RNs have revealed that about "40 percent of the 5,317 work shifts they logged exceeded twelve hours." Errors by hospital staff nurses are more likely to occur when work shifts extend beyond 12 hours, or they work over 40 hours in one week. Studies have shown that overtime shifts have harmful effects on the quality of care provided to patients, but some researchers "who evaluated the safety of 12-hour shifts did not find increases in medication errors." The errors which these researchers found were "lapses of attention to detail, errors of omission, compromised problem solving, reduced motivation" due to fatigue as well as "errors in grammatical reasoning and chart reviewing." Overworked nurses are a serious safety concern to their patients wellbeing. Working back to back shifts, or night shifts, are a common cause of fatigue in hospital staff nurses. "Less sleep, or fatigue, may lead to increased likelihood of making an error, or even the decreased likelihood of catching someone else's error." Limiting working hours and shift rotations could "reduce the adverse effects of fatigue" and increase the quality of care of patients.

Health Literacy

Health literacy is a common and serious safety concern. A study of 2,600 patients at two hospitals determined that between 26-60% of patients could not understand medication directions, a standard informed consent, or basic health care materials. This mismatch between a clinician's level of communication and a patient's ability to understand can lead to medication errors and adverse outcomes.

The Institute of Medicine (2004) report found low health literacy levels negatively affects healthcare outcomes. In particular, these patients have a higher risk of hospitalization and longer hospital stays, are less likely to comply with treatment, are more likely to make errors with medication, and are more ill when they seek medical care.

Pre-release Patient Education

Patients with irreversible airway compromise and bulbar paralysis due to various chronic, systemic and autoimmune diseases often have to continue with a lifelong tracheostomy. These patients require a cautious and meticulous home care of the tracheostomy tube and the stoma. Many centers and hospitals have their integrated pre-discharge patient education program and checklist. This is particularly mandatory and warrants due attention in regard of sending a patient home with a tracheostomy. A brief span hands-on training and comprehensive educational materials are to be ensured sincerely. It is vital to have/organize the support of relatives or a companion. At least one individual ought to learn how to help the patient in case of emergency. That person should join the patient when he/she gets guidelines in the hospital. Medical information and communication technology and digital modules should also be made easily accessible and user-friendly to the mass people.

Pay for Performance (P4P)

Pay for performance systems link compensation to measures of work quality or goals. As of 2005, 75 percent of all U.S. companies connect at least part of an employee's pay to measures of performance, and in healthcare, over 100 private and federal pilot programs are underway. Current methods of healthcare payment may actually reward less-safe care, since some insurance companies will not pay for new practices to reduce errors, while physicians and hospitals can bill for additional services that are needed when patients are injured by mistakes. However, early studies showed little gain in quality for the money spent, as well as evidence suggesting unintended consequences, like the avoidance of high-risk patients, when payment was linked to outcome improvements. The 2006 Institute of Medicine report *Preventing Medication Errors* recommended "incentives...so that profitability of hospitals, clinics, pharmacies, insurance companies, and manufacturers (are) aligned with patient safety goals;...(to) strengthen the business case for quality and safety."

There is widespread international interest in health care pay-for-performance programs in a range of countries, including the United Kingdom, United States, Australia, Canada, Germany, the Netherlands, and New Zealand.

United Kingdom

In the United Kingdom, the National Health Service (NHS) began an ambitious pay for performance initiative in 2004, known as the Quality and Outcomes Framework (QOF). General practitioners agreed to increases in existing income according to performance with respect to 146 quality indicators covering clinical care for 10 chronic diseases, organization of care, and patient experience. Unlike proposed quality incentive programs in the United States, funding for primary care was increased 20% over previous levels. This allowed practices to invest in extra staff and technology; 90% of general practitioners use the NHS Electronic Prescription Service, and up to 50% use electronic health records for the majority of clinical care. Early analysis showed that substantially increasing physicians' pay based on their success in meeting quality performance measures is successful. The 8,000 family practitioners included in the study earned an average of $40,000 more by collecting nearly 97% of the points available.

A component of this program, known as *exception reporting*, allows physicians to use criteria to exclude individual patients from the quality calculations that determine physician reimbursement. There was initial concern that exception reporting would allow inappropriate exclusion of patients in whom targets were missed ("gaming"). However, a 2008 study has shown little evidence of widespread gaming.

United States

In the United States, Medicare has various pay-for-performance ("P4P") initiatives in offices, clinics and hospitals, seeking to improving quality and avoid unnecessary health care costs. The Centers for Medicare and Medicaid Services (CMS) has several demonstration projects underway offering compensation for improvements:

- Payments for better care coordination between home, hospital and offices for patients with chronic illnesses. In April 2005, CMS launched its first value-based purchasing pilot or "demonstration" project- the three-year Medicare Physician Group Practice (PGP) Demonstration. The project involves ten large, multi-specialty physician practices caring for more than 200,000 Medicare fee-for-service beneficiaries. Participating practices will phase in quality standards for preventive care and the management of common chronic illnesses such as diabetes. Practices meeting these standards will be eligible for rewards from savings due to resulting improvements in patient management. The *First Evaluation Report to Congress* in 2006 showed that the model rewarded high quality, efficient provision of health care, but the lack of up-front payment for the investment in new systems of case management "have made for an uncertain future with respect for any payments under the demonstration."

- A set of 10 hospital quality measures which, if reported to CMS, will increase the payments that hospitals receive for each discharge. By the third year of the demonstration, those hospitals that do not meet a threshold on quality will be subject to reductions in payment. Preliminary data from the second year of the study indicates that pay for performance was associated with a roughly 2.5% to 4.0% improvement in compliance with quality measures, compared with the control hospitals. Dr. Arnold Epstein of the Harvard School of Public Health commented in an accompanying editorial that pay-for-performance "is fundamentally a social experiment likely to have only modest incremental value." Unintended consequences of some publicly reported hospital quality measures have adversely affected patient care. The requirement to give the first antibiotic dose in the emergency department within 4 hours, if the patient has pneumonia, has caused an increase in pneumonia misdiagnosis.

- Rewards to physicians for improving health outcomes by the use of health information technology in the care of chronically ill Medicare patients.

- Disincentives: The Tax Relief & Health Care Act of 2006 required the HHS Inspector General to study ways that Medicare payments to hospitals could be recouped for "never events", as defined by the National Quality Forum, including hospital infections. In August 2007, CMS announced that it will stop payments to hospitals for several negative consequences of care that result in injury, illness or death. This rule, effective October 2008, would reduce hospital payments for eight serious types of preventable incidents: objects left in a patient during surgery, blood transfusion reaction, air embolism, falls, mediastinitis, urinary tract infections from catheters, pressure ulcer, and sepsis from catheters. Reporting of "never events" and creation of performance benchmarks for hospitals are also mandated. Other private health payers are considering similar actions; in 2005, HealthPartners, a Minnesota health insurer, chose not to cover 27 types of "never events". The Leapfrog Group has announced that they will work with hospitals, health plans and consumer groups to advocate reducing payment for "never events", and will recognize hospitals that agree to certain steps when a serious avoidable adverse event occurs in the facility, including notifying the patient and patient safety organizations, and waiving costs. Physician groups involved in the management of complications, such as the Infectious Diseases Society of America, have voiced objections to these proposals, observing that "some patients develop infections despite application of all evidence-based practices known to avoid infection", and that a punitive response may discourage further study and slow the dramatic improvements that have already been made.

Complex Illness

Pay for performance programs often target patients with serious and complex illnesses; such patients commonly interact with multiple healthcare providers and facilities. However, pilot programs now underway focus on simple indicators such as improvement in lab values or use of emergency services, avoiding areas of complexity such as multiple complications or several treating specialists. A 2007 study analyzing Medicare beneficiaries' healthcare visits showed that a median of two primary care physicians and five specialists provide care for a single patient. The authors doubt that pay-for-performance systems can accurately attribute responsibility for the outcome of care for such patients. The American College of Physicians Ethics has stated concerns about using a limited set of clinical practice parameters to assess quality, "especially if payment for good performance is grafted onto the current payment system, which does not reward robust comprehensive care...The elderly patient with multiple chronic conditions is especially vulnerable to this unwanted effect of powerful incentives." Present pay-for-performance systems measure good performance based on specified clinical measurements, such as glycohemoglobin for diabetic patients. Healthcare providers who are monitored by such limited criteria have a powerful incentive to *deselect* (dismiss or refuse to accept) patients whose outcome measures fall below the quality standard and therefore worsen the provider's assessment. Patients with low health literacy, inadequate financial resources to afford expensive medications or treatments, and ethnic groups traditionally subject to healthcare inequities may also be deselected by providers seeking improved performance measures.

Public Reporting

Mandatory Reporting

Denmark

> The Danish Act on Patient Safety passed Parliament in June 2003, and on January 1, 2004, Denmark became the first country to introduce nationwide mandatory reporting. The Act obligates frontline personnel to report adverse events to a national reporting system. Hospital owners are obligated to act on the reports and the National Board of Health is obligated to communicate the learning nationally. The reporting system is intended purely for learning and frontline personnel cannot experience sanctions for reporting. This is stated in Section 6 of the Danish Act on Patient Safety (as of January 1, 2007: Section 201 of the Danish Health Act): "A frontline person who reports an adverse event cannot as a result of that report be subjected to investigation or disciplinary action from the employer, the Board of Health or the Court of Justice." The reporting system and the Danish Patient Safety Database is described in further detail in a National Board of Health publication.

United Kingdom

> The National Patient Safety Agency encourages voluntary reporting of health care errors, but has several specific instances, known as "Confidential Enquiries", for which investigation is routinely initiated: maternal or infant deaths, childhood deaths to age 16, deaths in persons with mental illness, and perioperative and unexpected medical deaths. Medical records and questionnaires are requested from the involved clinician, and participation has been high, since individual details are confidential.

United States

> The 1999 Institute of Medicine (IOM) report recommended "a nationwide mandatory reporting system ... that provides for ... collection of standardized information by state governments about adverse events that result in death or serious harm." Professional organizations, such as the Anesthesia Patient Safety Foundation, responded negatively: "Mandatory reporting systems in general create incentives for individuals and institutions

to play a numbers game. If such reporting becomes linked to punitive action or inappropriate public disclosure, there is a high risk of driving reporting "underground", and of reinforcing the cultures of silence and blame that many believe are at the heart of the problems of medical error..."

Although 23 states established mandatory reporting systems for serious patient injuries or death by 2005, the national database envisioned in the IOM report was delayed by the controversy over mandatory versus voluntary reporting. Finally in 2005, the US Congress passed the long-debated Patient Safety and Quality Improvement Act, establishing a federal reporting database. Hospitals reports of serious patient harm are voluntary, collected by patient safety organizations under contract to analyze errors and recommend improvements. The federal government serves to coordinate data collection and maintain the national database. Reports remain confidential, and cannot be used in liability cases. Consumer groups have objected to the lack of transparency, claiming it denies the public information on the safety of specific hospitals.

Individual Patient Disclosures

For a health care institution, disclosing an unanticipated event should be made as soon as possible. Some health care organizations may have a policy regarding the disclosure of unanticipated events. The amount of information presented to those affected is dependent on the family's readiness and the organization's culture. The employee disclosing the event to family requires support from risk management, patient safety officers and senior leadership. Disclosures are objectively documented in the medical record.

Voluntary Disclosure

In public surveys, a significant majority of those surveyed believe that health care providers should be required to report all serious medical errors publicly. However, reviews of the medical literature show little effect of publicly reported performance data on patient safety or the quality of care. Public reporting on the quality of individual providers or hospitals does not seem to affect selection of hospitals and individual providers. Some studies have shown that reporting performance data stimulates quality improvement activity in hospitals.

United States

Medical Error

Ethical standards of the Joint Commission on Accreditation of Healthcare Organizations (JCAHO), the American Medical Association (AMA) Council on Ethical and Judicial Affairs, and the American College of Physicians Ethics Manual require disclosure of the most serious adverse events. However, many doctors and hospitals do not report errors under the current system because of concerns about malpractice lawsuits; this prevents collection of information needed to find and correct the conditions that lead to mistakes. As of 2008, 35 US states have statutes allowing doctors and health care providers to apologize and offer expressions of regret without their words being used against them in court, and 7 states have also passed laws mandating written disclosure of adverse events and bad outcomes to patients and families. In September 2005, US Senators

Clinton and Obama introduced the National Medical Error Disclosure and Compensation (MED-iC) Bill, providing physicians protection from liability and a safe environment for disclosure, as part of a program to notify and compensate patients harmed by medical errors. It is now the policy of several academic medical centers, including Johns Hopkins, University of Illinois and Stanford, to promptly disclose medical errors, offering apologies and compensation. This national initiative, hoping to restore integrity to dealings with patients, make it easier to learn from mistakes and avoid angry lawsuits, was modeled after a University of Michigan Hospital System program that has reduced the number of lawsuits against the hospital by 75% and has decreased the average litigation cost. The Veterans Health Administration requires the disclosure of all adverse events to patients, even those that are not obvious. However, as of 2008 these initiatives have only included hospitals that are self-insured and that employ their staffs, thus limiting the number of parties involved. Medical errors are the third leading cause of death in the US, after heart disease and cancer, according to research by Johns Hopkins University. Their study published in May 2016 concludes that more than 250,000 people die every year due to medical mix-ups. Other countries report similar results.

Performance

In April 2008, consumer, employer and labor organizations announced an agreement with major physician organizations and health insurers on principles to measure and report doctors' performance on quality and cost.

United Kingdom

In the United Kingdom, whistleblowing is well recognised and is government sanctioned, as a way to protect patients by encouraging employees to call attention to deficient services. Health authorities are encouraged to put local policies in place to protect whistleblowers.

Studies of Patient Safety

Numerous organizations, government branches, and private companies conduct research studies to investigate the overall health of patient safety in America and across the globe. Despite the shocking and widely publicized statistics on preventable deaths due to medical errors in America's hospitals, the 2006 National Healthcare Quality Report assembled by the Agency for Healthcare Research and Quality (AHRQ) had the following sobering assessment:

- Most measures of Quality are improving, but the pace of change remains modest.

- Quality improvement varies by setting and phase of care.

- The rate of improvement accelerated for some measures while a few continued to show deterioration.

- Variation in health care quality remains high.

A 2011 study of more than 1,000 patients with advanced colon cancer found that one in eight was treated with at least one drug regimen with specific recommendations against their use in the National Comprehensive Cancer Network guidelines. The study focused on three chemotherapy regimens that were not supported by evidence from prior clinical studies or clinical practice guidelines. One treatment was rated "insufficient data to support," one had been "shown to be ineffective," and one was supported by "no data, nor is there a compelling rationale." Many of the patients received multiple cycles of non-beneficial chemotherapy and some received two or more unproven treatments. Potential side effects for the treatments include hypertension, heightened risk of bleeding and bowel perforation.

Organizations Advocating Patient Safety

Several authors of the 1999 Institute of Medicine report revisited the status of their recommendations and the state of patient safety, five years after "To Err is Human". Discovering that patient safety had become a frequent topic for journalists, health care experts, and the public, it was harder to see overall improvements on a national level. What was noteworthy was the impact on attitudes and organizations. Few health care professionals now doubted that preventable medical injuries were a serious problem. The central concept of the report—that bad systems and not bad people lead to most errors—became established in patient safety efforts. A broad array of organizations now advance the cause of patient safety. For instance, in 2010 the principal European anaesthesiology organisations launched The Helsinki Declaration for Patient Safety in Anaesthesiology, which incorporates many of the principles described above.

Team Nursing

Team nursing is a system of integrated care that was developed in 1950s (under grant from W.K. Kellogg Foundation) directed by Eleanor Lambertson at Teachers College, Columbia University in New York, NY. Because the functional method received criticism, a new system of nursing was devised to improve patient satisfaction. "Care through others" became the hallmark of team nursing. It was developed in an effort to decrease the problems associated with the functional model of nursing care. Many people felt that, despite a continued shortage of professional nursing staff, a patient care delivery model had to be developed that reduced the fragmented care that accompanies functional nursing.

Team nursing was developed because of social and technological changes in World War II drew many nurses away from hospitals, learning haps, services, procedures and equipment became more expensive and complicated, requiring specialisation at every turn. It is an attempt to meet increased demands of nursing services and better use of knowledge and skills of professional nurses.

Definitions

- Team nursing is a system that distributes the care of a patient amongst a team that is all working together to provide for this person. This team consists of up to 4 to 6 members that has a team leader who gives jobs and instructions to the group.

- Team nursing is based on philosophy in which groups of professional and non-professional personnel work together to identify, plan, implement and evaluate comprehensive client-centered care. The key concept is a group that works together toward a common goal, providing qualitative, comprehensive nursing care.Team nursing was designed to accommodate several categories of personnel in meeting the comprehensive nursing needs of a group of clients

Objective

The objective of team nursing is to give the best possible quality of patient care by utilising the abilities of every member of the staff to the fullest extent and by providing close supervision both of patient care and of the individual who give it.

Line of Organisation

A clear line of organisation structure is needed for team nursing to provide a mechanism for horizontal and vertical communication, and an organised pattern is employed.

Functions

The two important points of functioning are:

1. The head nurse must know at all times the condition of the patients and the plan for their care and must be assured that assignments and workmanship contribute to quality nursing

2. The team leader must have freedom to use their initiative and the opportunity to nurse, supervise, and teach unencumbered by the responsibility for administrative detail

Functions of a Registered Nurse

- In team nursing the registered nurse (RN) functions as a team leader, and coordinates the small group (no more than four or five) of ancillary personnel to provide care to a small group of patients.

- As coordinator of the team, the RN must know the many conditions and needs of all patients assigned to the team and plan for the individualised care for each patient.

- The team leader is also responsible for encouraging a cooperative environment and maintaining clear communication among all team members.

- The team leader's duties include planning care, assigning duties, directing and assisting team members, giving direct patient care, teaching and coordinating patient activities.

- The team leader assigns each member specific responsibilities dependent on the role.

- The members of the team report directly to the team leader, who then reports to the charge nurse or unit manager.

- Communication is enhanced through the use of written patient assignments, the development of nursing care plans, and the use of regularly scheduled team conferences to discuss the patient status and formulate revisions to the plan of care.

- However, for team nursing to succeed, the team leader must have strong clinical skills, good communication skills, delegation ability, decision-making ability, and the ability to create a cooperative working environment.^

Channels of Communication

1. Reports

2. Work or assignment conference

3. Patient care conference

4. Written nursing care plan

The greatest single distinguishing feature of team nursing is the team conference. In general, there are three parts to the conference;

- Report by each team member on his or her patients.

- Planning for new patients and changing plans as needed for others.

- Planning the next day's assessment.

It is essential that the conference be well planned, brief but comprehensive and interesting. The team leader is the chair person for the conference. They offer opportunity for all personnel to evaluate patient care and solve the problems through team discussion.

Advantages:

1. High quality comprehensive care can be provided despite a relatively high proportion of ancillary staff.

2. Each member of the team is able to participate in decision making and problem solving.

3. Each team member is able to contribute his or her own special expertise or skills in caring for the patient.

4. Improved patient satisfaction.

5. Organisational decision making occurring at the lower level.

6. Cost-effective system because it works with expected ratio of unlicensed to licensed personnel.

7. Team nursing is an effective method of patient care delivery and has been used in most inpatient and outpatient health care settings.

Other advantages:

1. Feeling of participation and belonging are facilitated with team members.

2. Work load can be balanced and shared.

3. Division of labour allows members the opportunity to develop leadership skills.

4. Every team member has the opportunity to learn from and teach colleagues

5. There is a variety in the daily assignment.

6. Interest in client's wellbeing and care is shared by several people, reliability of decisions is increased.

7. Nursing care hours are usually cost effective.

8. The client is able to identify personnel who are responsible for his care.

9. Continuity of care is facilitated, especially if teams are constant.

10. Barriers between professional and non-professional workers can be minimised, the group efforts prevail.

11. Everyone has the opportunity to contribute to the care plan.

Disadvantages:

1. Establishing a team concept takes time, effort and constancy of personnel. Merely assigning people to a group does not make them a 'group' or 'team'.

2. Unstable staffing pattern make team nursing difficult.

3. All personnel must be client centred.

4. There is less individual responsibility and independence regarding nursing functions.

5. Continuity of care may suffer if the daily team assignments vary and the patient is confronted with many different caregivers.

6. The team leader may not have the leadership skills required to effectively direct the team and create a "team spirit".

7. Insufficient time for care planning and communication may lead to unclear goals. Therefore, responsibilities and care may become fragmented.

Modifications: In an attempt to overcome some of its disadvantages, the team nursing design has been modified many times since its original inception, and variations of the model are evident in other methods of nursing care delivery such, as modular nursing.

Modular Nursing

Modular nursing is a modification of team nursing and focuses on the patient's geographic location for staff assignments.

- The patient unit is divided into modules or districts, and the same team of caregivers is assigned consistently to the same geographic location.

- Each location, or module, has an RN assigned as the team leader, and the other team members may include LVN/LPN or UAP.

- Just as in the team nursing, the team leader in the modular nursing is accountable for all patient care and is responsible for providing leadership for team members and creating a cooperative work environment.

- The concept of modular nursing calls for a smaller group of staff providing care for a smaller group of patients.

- The goal is to increase the involvement of the RN in planning and coordinating care.

- Communication is more efficient among a smaller group of team members.

- The success of the modular nursing depends greatly on the leadership abilities of the team leader.

Advantages:

1. Continuity of care is improved when staff members are consistently assigned to the same module

2. The RN as team leader is able to be more involved in planning and coordinating care.

3. Geographic closeness and more efficient communication save staff time.

Disadvantages:

1. Costs may be increased to stock each module with the necessary patient care supplies (medication cart, linens and dressings).

2. Long corridors, common in many hospitals, are not conducive to modular nursing.

Nurse Scheduling Problem

The nurse scheduling problem (NSP), also called the nurse rostering problem (NRP), is the operations research problem of finding an optimal way to assign nurses to shifts, typically with a set of hard constraints which all valid solutions must follow, and a set of soft constraints which define the relative quality of valid solutions. Solutions to the nurse scheduling problem can be applied to constrained scheduling problems in other fields.

The nurse scheduling problem has been studied since before 1969, and is known to have NP-hard complexity.

General Description

The nurse scheduling problem involves the assignment of shifts and holidays to nurses. Each nurse has their own wishes and restrictions, as does the hospital. The problem is described as finding a schedule that both respects the constraints of the nurses and fulfills the objectives of the hospital. Conventionally, a nurse can work 3 shifts because nursing is shift work:

- day shift

- night shift

- late night shift

In this problem we must search for a solution satisfying as many wishes as possible while not compromising the needs of the hospital.

Constraints

There are two types of constraints:

- hard constraints: if this constraint fails then the entire schedule is invalid.

- soft constraints: it is desirable that these constraints are met but not meeting them doesn't make the schedule invalid.

Some examples of constraints are:

- A nurse doesn't work the day shift, night shift and late night shift on the same day (for obvious reasons).

- A nurse may go on a holiday and will not work shifts during this time.

- A nurse doesn't do a late night shift followed by a day shift the next day.

Hard constraints typically include a specification of shifts (e.g. morning, afternoon, and night), that each nurse should work no more than one shift per day, and that all patients should have nursing coverage. Differences in qualifications between nurses also create hard constraints. Soft constraints may include minimum and maximum numbers of shifts assigned to a given nurse in a given week, of hours worked per week, of days worked consecutively, of days off consecutively, and so on. The shift preferences of individual nurses may be treated as a soft constraint, or as a hard constraint.

Solutions

Solutions to the problem use a variety of techniques, including both mathematically exact solutions and a variety of heuristic solutions using decomposition, parallel computing, stochastic optimization, genetic algorithms, colony optimization, simulated annealing, Tabu search, and coordinate descent.

Burke *et al.* (2004) summarised the state of art of academic research to the nurse rostering problem, including brief introductions of various then published solutions.

Nurse–client Relationship

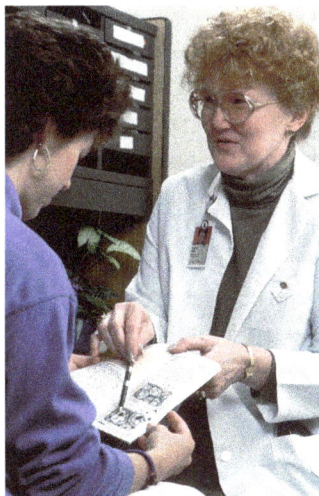

Nurse explaining information in a brochure with a client. Picture was taken by Bill Branson (Photographer).

The nurse–client relationship is an interaction aimed to enhance the well-being of a "client," which may be an individual, a family, a group, or a community. Peplau's theory is of high relevance to the nurse-client relationship, with one of its major aspects being that both the nurse and the client become more knowledgeable and mature over the course of their relationship. Peplau believed that the relationship depended on the interaction of the thoughts, feelings, and actions of each person and that the patient will experience better health when all their specific needs are fully considered in the relationship.

Elements

The nurse-client relationship is composed of several elements.

Boundaries

Boundaries are an integral part of the nurse-client relationship. They represent invisible structures imposed by legal, ethical, and professional standards of nursing that respect the rights of nurses and clients. These boundaries ensure that the focus of the relationship remains on the client's needs, not only by word but also by law. The College of Nurses of Ontario (CNO) Standards identifies that it is the nurse's responsibility to establish the boundaries and limits of the relationship between the nurse and client. The boundaries have a specific purpose and health goal, and the relationship terminates when identified goal is met.

Any action or behaviour in a nurse-client relationship that personally benefits the nurse at the expense of the client is a boundary violation. Some examples of boundary violations are engaging in a romantic or sexual relationship with a current client, extensive non-beneficial disclosure to the client and receiving a gift of money from the client. Abuse and neglect are extreme examples. They involve the betrayal of respect and trust within the relationship. This includes withholding communication from a client because it is considered to be an example of neglect.

It is the nurse's job to be aware of signs that professional boundaries may be crossed or have been crossed. Warning signs of boundary crossing that may lead to boundary violations include frequently thinking of a client in a personal way, keeping secrets with a specific client, favouring one client's care at the expense of another's and telling a client personal things about yourself in order to make an impression. Anything that could comprise the client's well-being if the relationship with a registered nurse is continued or discontinued can be considered a warning sign. Boundary violations are never acceptable and it is the nurse's job to handle any situation with any regards to it professionally and therapeutically regardless of who initiated it.

Confidentiality

This makes the relationship safe and establishes trust. The patient should feel comfortable disclosing personal information and asking questions. The nurse is to share information only with professional staff that needs to know and obtain the client's written permission to share information with others outside the treatment team.

Therapeutic Nurse Behaviours

Nurses are expected to always act in the best interests of the patient to maintain a relationship that is strictly with all intent to only benefit the client. The nurse must ensure that their client's needs are met while being professional. Extensive research and clinical observation has shown that the body, mind and emotions are in unity. Therefore, in order to help another person, one must consider all these aspects; this means not neglecting the person and strictly just treating the illness. Caring for patients is beyond the treatment of disease and disability.

The necessary knowledge aspects that are needed to maintain a therapeutic nurse-client relationship are: background knowledge, knowledge of interpersonal and development theory, knowledge of diversity influences and determinants, knowledge of person, knowledge of health/illness, knowledge of the broad influences on health care and health care policy, and knowledge of systems.

Background knowledge is the nurse's education, and her life experience. Knowledge of interpersonal and development theory is the knowledge of theories of the sense of self and self influence on others. The specific theories are: The Interpersonal Theory, Object relation theory, Developmental theory, and Gender/developmental theory. Knowledge of person explains that nurses must take the time to understand the client, and their world; what is meaningful to them, and their history. Knowledge of Health and Illness is the knowledge that the nurse must attain about their client's health issue. Knowledge of the broad influences on health care and health care policy explains that nurses need to be aware of the influences of the client's care; social/political forces, expectations of health-care system, and changes in accessibility, and resources. Knowledge of Systems explains that the nurse needs to know about the health-care system so they can help their clients access services. Effective communication in nursing entails being empathic, non-judgmental, understanding, approachable, sympathetic, caring, and having safe and ethical qualities. The first statement of the CNO Standard is Therapeutic Communication, which explains that a nurse should apply communication and interpersonal skills to create, maintain, and terminate a nurse-client relationship.

All of the aspects to a therapeutic relationship are interrelated. You cannot efficiently use one aspect without the other; they are all connected and work together to create a successful relationship. Nurses assist clients to achieve their health related goals including improving their relationship with others. "The help that nurses offer to their clients is much more than technical expertise. The relationship between nurse and client is a powerful healing force by itself.

Self-awareness

Self-awareness is an internal evaluation of one self and of one's reactions to emotionally charged situations, people and places. It offers an opportunity to recognize how our attitudes, perceptions, past and present experiences, and relationships frame or distort interactions with others. An example of self-awareness would be acknowledging that showing anger is not a sign of weakness, because there were emotions outside of your control. Self-awareness allows you to fully engage with a client and presence; being with the client in the moment, allows the nurse to know when to provide help and when to stand back. Until individuals can fully understand themselves they cannot understand others. Nurses need self-awareness in this relationship to be able to relate to the patient's experiences to develop empathy.

Genuine, Warm and Respectful

Highly skilled, experienced nurses must possessed certain attributes or skills to successfully establish a nurse client relationship. Attributes such as being genuine, warm and respectful are a few to mention. An aspect of respect is respecting an individual's culture and ensuring open-mindedness is being incorporated all throughout the relationship up until the termination phase. The nurse works to empower the client along with their family to get more engaged in learning about their health and ways in which it can be improved. It is highly beneficial for the client to incorporate their family, as they may be the most effective support system. Revealing your whole self and being genuine with clients will accomplish the desired nurse client relationship.

Behaving therapeutically may require remaining silent at times to display acceptance, incorporating open ended questions to allow the client control of the conversation and encouragement to continue. In addition, the nurse may also reduce distance to demonstrate their desire in being involved, restating and reflecting to validate the nurse's interpretation of the client's message, directing the conversation towards important topics by focusing in on them. Nurses also seek clarification to demonstrate the desire to understand, summarizing to help aid the client in separating the relevant information from the irrelevant ones. Nurses must make their client feel confidant that they will be treated courteously and that their nurses show genuine interest in them.

The strong connections between clients and nurses are made by presence, touch and listening. Furthermore, being polite and punctual displays respect for the client in addition to remembering to be patient, understanding, also to praise and encourage the client for their attempts to take better care of their health. A primary factor in establishing a nurse client relationship is the non-verbal message or behaviours you send out unconsciously, resulting in a negative perception and may distort your attempts in effectively assisting the client to achieve optimal health. One of the non-verbal factors is listening. Listening behaviours are identified as S.O.L.E.R; S-sit squarely in relation to client, O-maintain an open position and do not cross arms or legs, L-lean slightly towards the client, E-maintain reasonable and comfortable eye contact, R-relax. These behaviours are effective for communication skills, and are useful for thinking about how to listen to another person.

Empathy

Having the ability to enter the perceptual world of the other person and understanding how they experience the situation is empathy. This is an important therapeutic nurse behaviour essential to convey support, understanding and share experiences. A client to a nurse in a general sense is seeking help. Patients are expecting a nurse who will show interest, sympathy, and an understanding of their difficulties. When receiving care patients tend to be looking for more than the treatment of their disease or disability, they want to receive psychological consideration. This happens through good communication, communication with clients is the foundation of care.

During hard times, clients are looking for a therapeutic relationship that will make their treatment as less challenging as possible. Many patients are aware that a solution to their problems may not be available but expect to have support through them and that this is what defines a positive or negative experience. Empathy is used as a tool to enhance the communication between the nurse and client. Past experiences can help the clinician can better understand issues in order to provide better intervention and treatment.

Cultural Sensitivity

Healthcare is a multicultural environment and nurses have to expect that they will care for patients from many different culture and ethical backgrounds. Cultural backgrounds effect people's perceptions of life and health. The goal of the nurse is to develop a body of knowledge that allows them to provide cultural specific care. This begins with an open mind and accepting attitude.

Cultural competence is a viewpoint that increases respect and awareness for patients from cultures different from the nurse's own. Cultural sensitivity is putting aside our own perspective to understand another person's perceptive. Caring and culture are described as being intricately linked. This is believed because there can be no cure without caring and caring involves knowing the different values and behaviours of a person's culture. It is important to assess language needs and request for a translation service if needed and provide written material in the patient's language. As well as, trying to mimic the patient's style of communication (e.g. little direct eye contact, slow, quiet).

A major obstacle to cultural sensitivity and good communication is ethnocentrism, which is the belief that ones ethical group is superior to another; this causes prejudice and stops a nurse for fully understanding the patient. Another obstacle is stereotyping, a patient's background is often multifaceted encompassing many ethic and cultural traditions. In order to individualize communication and provide culturally sensitive care it is important to understand the complexity of social, ethnic, cultural and economic. This involves overcoming certain attitudes and offering consistent, non-judgemental care to all patients. Accepting the person for who they are regardless of diverse backgrounds and circumstances or differences in morals or beliefs. By exhibiting these attributes trust can grow between patient and nurse. Nurses need to know the outcome of social, cultural, and racial differences, and how they can affect the therapeutic relationship. Nurses need to acknowledge the impact of culture in order to practice health in a way that respects a person's beliefs and values.

Collaborative Goal Setting

A therapeutic nurse-client relationship is established for the benefit of the client. It includes nurses working with the client to create goals directed at improving their health status. Goals are centered on the client's values, beliefs and needs. A partnership is formed between nurse and client. The nurse empowers patient and families to get involved in their health. This relationship has three phases, a beginning (first time contact/introduction), a middle (develop a relationship to deliver care) and an end (the patient is no longer dependant on the nurse). To make this process successful the nurse must value, respect and listen to clients as individuals. Focus should be on the feelings, priorities, challenges, and ideas of the patient, with progressive aim of enhancing optimum physical, spiritual, and mental health.

Responsible, Ethical Practice

This is a communication-based relationship, therefore, a responsibility to interact, educate, and share information genuinely is placed upon the nurse. The fourth statement of the CNO Standard is, Protecting Clients from Abuse. It is stated that it is the nurse's job to report abuse of their client to ensure that their client is safe from harm. Nurses must intervene and report any abusive situations observed that might be seen as violent, threatening, or intended to inflict harm. Nurses must also report any health care provider's behaviors or remarks towards clients that are perceived as romantic, or sexually abusive.

Clients' Perspectives

Coatsworth-Puspoky, Forchuk, and Ward-Griffin conducted a study on clients' perspectives in the nurse–client relationship. Interviews were done with participants from Southern Ontario, ten had been hospitalized for a psychiatric illness and four had experiences with nurses from community-based organizations, but were never hospitalized. The participants were asked about experiences at different stages of the relationship. The research described two relationships that formed the "bright side" and the "dark side".

The "bright" relationship involved nurses who validated clients and their feelings. For example, one client tested his trust of the nurse by becoming angry with her and revealing his negative thoughts related to the hospitalization. The client stated, "she's trying to be quite nice to me ... if she's able to tolerate this occasional venomous attack, which she has done quite well right up to now, it will probably be a very beneficial relationship".

The "dark" side of the relationship resulted in the nurse and client moving away from each other. For example, one client stated, "The nurses' general feeling was when someone asks for help, they're being manipulative and attention seeking". The nurse didn't recognize the client who has an illness with needs therefore; the clients avoided the nurse and perceived the nurse as avoiding them. One patient reported, "the nurses all stayed in their central station. They didn't mix with the patients ... The only interaction you have with them is medication time". Neither trust nor caring was exchanged so perceptions of mutual avoiding and ignoring resulted. One participant stated, "no one cares. It doesn't matter. It's just, they don't want to hear it. They don't want to know it; they don't want to listen". The relationship that developed depended on the nurse's personality and attitude. These findings bring awareness about the importance of the nurse–client relationship.

Building Trust

Building trust is beneficial to how the relationship progresses. Wiesman used interviews with 15 participants who spent at least three days in intensive care to investigate the factors that helped develop trust in the nurse–client relationship. Patients said nurses promoted trust through attentiveness, competence, comfort measures, personality traits, and provision of information. Every participant stated the attentiveness of the nurse was important to develop trust. One said the nurses "are with you all the time. Whenever anything comes up, they're in there caring for you". Competence was seen by seven participants as being important in the development of trust. "I trusted the nurses because I could see them doing their job. They took time to do little things and made sure they were done right and proper," stated one participant. The relief of pain was seen by five participants as promoting trust.

One client stated, "they were there for the smallest need. I remember one time where they repositioned me maybe five or six times in a matter of an hour". A good personality was stated by five participants as important. One said, "they were all friendly, and they make you feel like they've known you for a long time" (61). Receiving adequate information was important to four participants. One participant said, "they explained things. They followed it through, step by step". The findings of this study show how trust is beneficial to a lasting relationship.

Emotional Support

Emotional Support is giving and receiving reassurance and encouragement done through understanding. Yamashita, Forchuk, and Mound conducted a study to examine the process of nurse case management involving clients with mental illness. Nurses in inpatient, transitional, and community settings in four cities in Ontario Canada were interviewed. The interviews show the importance of providing emotional support to the patients. One nurse stated that if the client knows "Somebody really cares enough to see how they are doing once a week ... by going shopping with them or to a doctor's appointment. To them it means the world".

The interviews showed it was crucial to include the family as therapeutic allies. A nurse stated that "We're with the families. We can be with them as oppositional and overly involved and somewhere else in between, and we're in contact with them as much as they want". With frequent contact the nurse was able to discuss possibilities with the family. The study reaffirmed the importance of emotional support in the relationship.

Humour

Humour is important in developing a lasting relationship. Astedt-Kurki, Isola, Tammentie, and Kervinen asked readers to write about experiences with humour while in the hospital through a patient organization newsletter. Letters were chosen from 13 chronically ill clients from Finland. The clients were also interviewed in addition to their letters. The interviews reported that humour played an important role in health. A paralyzed woman said, "Well you have to have a sense of humour if you want to live and survive. You have to keep it up no matter how much it hurts".

Humour helped clients accept what happened by finding a positive outlook. One participant stated, "... when you're sick as you can be and do nothing but lie down and another person does everything in her power to help, humour really makes you feel good". Humour also serves as a defence mechanism, especially in men. A participant said, "For male patients humour is also a way of concealing their feelings. It's extremely hard for them to admit they're afraid". The patient finds it easier to discuss difficult matters when a nurse has a sense of humour. "A nurse who has a sense of humour, ... that's the sort of nurse you can talk to, that's the sort of nurse you can turn to and ask for help ..." reported a participant. This study lends support that if humour is generally important to people, then in times of change it will remain important.

References

- Houweling, Lynn (2004). "Image, function, and style: A history of the nursing uniform.". American Journal of Nursing: American Journal of Nursing. 104 (4): 40–8. PMID 15171114

- "NCI Dictionary of Cancer Terms". National Cancer Institute. U.S. Department of Health and Human Services. Retrieved 12 January 2017

- Patrick A. Palmieri; et al. (2008). "The anatomy and physiology of error in averse healthcare events". Advances in Health Care Management. 7: 33–68. doi:10.1016/S1474-8231(08)07003-1

- Wong, F.K.; Chung, L.C. (2006). "Establishing a definition for a nurse-led clinic: structure, process, and outcome". Journal of Advanced Nursing. 53 (3): 358–369. PMID 16441541. doi:10.1111/j.1365-2648.2006.03730

- Kohn, Linda T.; Corrigan, Janet M.; Donaldson, Molla S., eds. (2000). To Err is Human—Building a Safer Health System. Washington, D. C.: National Academies Press. p. 312. ISBN 978-0-309-06837-6

- Ndosi, M; Vinall, K; Hale, C; Bird, H; Hill, J (2011). "The effectiveness of nurse-led care in people with rheumatoid arthritis: A systematic review". Int. J. Nurs. Stud. 48 (5): 642–54. doi:10.1016/j.ijnurstu.2011.02.007

- "Standards of Medical Care in Diabetes". Diabetes Professional Resources Online. American Diabetes Association. Retrieved 12 January 2017

- Wirth, Stephen. "Pro Bono: Stay Current on EMS Standards of Care to Avoid Liability Risk". Journal of Emergency Medical Services. PennWell Corporation. Retrieved 12 January 2017

- Frank JR, Brien S (August 2009). "The Safety Competencies - Enhancing Patient Safety Across the Health Professions" (PDF) (first ed.). Canadian Patient Safety Institute. ISBN 978-1-926541-15-0

- "Clinical Guidelines, Standards & Quality of Care". New York State. New York Department of Health. Retrieved 12 January 2017

- Weingart SN, Wilson RM, Gibberd RW, Harrison B (March 2000). "Epidemiology of medical error". BMJ. 320 (7237): 774–7. PMC 1117772. PMID 10720365. doi:10.1136/bmj.320.7237.774

- Neale, G; Woloshynowych, M; Vincent, C (July 2001). "Exploring the causes of adverse events in NHS hospital practice". Journal of the Royal Society of Medicine. 94 (7): 322–30. PMC 1281594. PMID 11418700

- Department of Health Expert Group (2000). "An organisation with a memory". Department of Health, United Kingdom. Retrieved 2006-07-01

- Committee on the Work Environment for Nurses and Patient Safety, Board of Health Care Services, Institute of Medicine (Feb 27, 2004). Page, Ann, ed. Keeping Patients Safe: Transforming the Work Environment of Nurses. National Academics Press. p. 12. ISBN 0309187362

- Kaushal, R; Bates, DW; et al. (2001). "Medication errors and adverse drug events in pediatric inpatients". JAMA. 285 (16): 2114–20. doi:10.1001/jama.285.16.2114

- "Incorporating Patient-Safe Design into the Guidelines". The American Institute of Architects Academy Journal. The American Institute of Architects. 2005-10-19

- David Marx. "Patient Safety and the "Just Culture:" A Primer For Health Care Executives" (PDF). University of California Los Angeles. Retrieved 30 October 2014

- Kessler, JM (Winter 2005). "Pharmacy Quality Assurance". Journal of the North Carolina Association of Pharmacists

- National Quality Forum (2007). Serious Reportable Events in Healthcare 2006 Update: A Consensus Report. Washington, D.C.: National Quality Forum. ISBN 1-933875-08-9. Retrieved 2007-08-25

- Miller, MR; Elixhauser, A; Zhan, C (June 2003). "Patient safety events during pediatric hospitalizations". Pediatrics. 111 (6): 1358–66. doi:10.1542/peds.111.6.1358

5

Health Care: An Essential Aspect

Health care is concerned with the diagnosis, treatment and prevention of illnesses, injuries and disorders. It encompasses professional health care services as well as care provided at the home. It varies from country to country and mainly depends on the economical condition of the nation. This chapter is an overview of the subject matter incorporating all the major aspects of health care.

Health Care

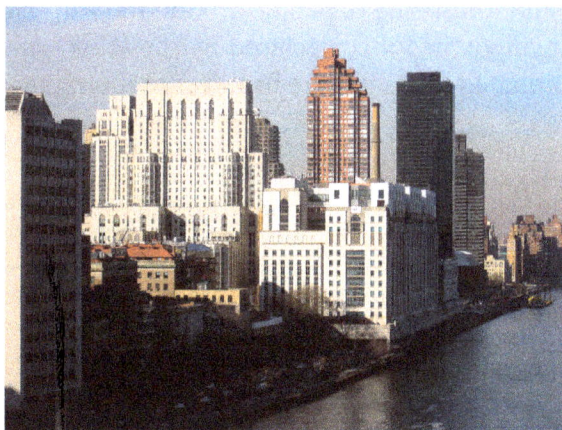

New York-Presbyterian Hospital in New York City is one of the world's busiest hospitals. Pictured is the Weill-Cornell facility (white complex at centre).

Health care or healthcare is the maintenance or improvement of health via the diagnosis, treatment, and prevention of disease, illness, injury, and other physical and mental impairments in human beings. Healthcare is delivered by health professionals (providers or practitioners) in allied health professions, chiropractic, physicians, physician associates, dentistry, midwifery, nursing, medicine, optometry, pharmacy, psychology, and other health professions. It includes the work done in providing primary care, secondary care, and tertiary care, as well as in public health.

Access to healthcare varies across countries, groups, and individuals, largely influenced by social and economic conditions as well as the health policies in place. Countries and jurisdictions have different policies and plans in relation to the personal and population-based health care goals within their societies. Healthcare systems are organizations established to meet the health needs of target populations. Their exact configuration varies between national and subnational entities. In some countries and jurisdictions, healthcare planning is distributed among market participants, whereas in others, planning occurs more centrally among governments or other coordinating bodies. In all cases, according to the World Health Organization (WHO), a well-functioning healthcare system requires a robust financing mechanism; a well-trained and adequately-paid workforce;

reliable information on which to base decisions and policies; and well maintained health facilities and logistics to deliver quality medicines and technologies.

Healthcare can contribute to a significant part of a country's economy. In 2011, the healthcare industry consumed an average of 9.3 percent of the GDP or US$ 3,322 (PPP-adjusted) per capita across the 34 members of OECD countries. The USA (17.7%, or US$ PPP 8,508), the Netherlands (11.9%, 5,099), France (11.6%, 4,118), Germany (11.3%, 4,495), Canada (11.2%, 5669), and Switzerland (11%, 5,634) were the top spenders, however life expectancy in total population at birth was highest in Switzerland (82.8 years), Japan and Italy (82.7), Spain and Iceland (82.4), France (82.2) and Australia (82.0), while OECD's average exceeds 80 years for the first time ever in 2011: 80.1 years, a gain of 10 years since 1970. The USA (78.7 years) ranges only on place 26 among the 34 OECD member countries, but has the highest costs by far. All OECD countries have achieved universal (or almost universal) health coverage, except Mexico and the USA.

Healthcare is conventionally regarded as an important determinant in promoting the general physical and mental health and well-being of people around the world. An example of this was the worldwide eradication of smallpox in 1980, declared by the WHO as the first disease in human history to be completely eliminated by deliberate health care interventions.

Delivery

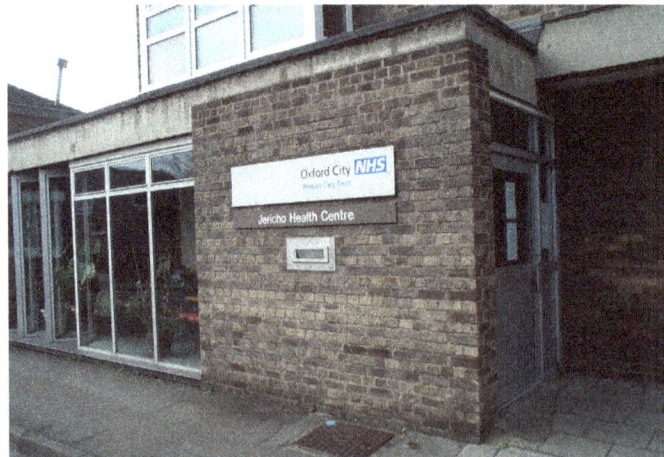

Primary care may be provided in community health centres

The delivery of modern health care depends on groups of trained professionals and paraprofessionals coming together as interdisciplinary teams. This includes professionals in medicine, psychology, physiotherapy, nursing, dentistry, midwifery and allied health, plus many others such as public health practitioners, community health workers and assistive personnel, who systematically provide personal and population-based preventive, curative and rehabilitative care services.

While the definitions of the various types of health care vary depending on the different cultural, political, organizational and disciplinary perspectives, there appears to be some consensus that primary care constitutes the first element of a continuing health care process, that may also include the provision of secondary and tertiary levels of care. Healthcare can be defined as either public or private.

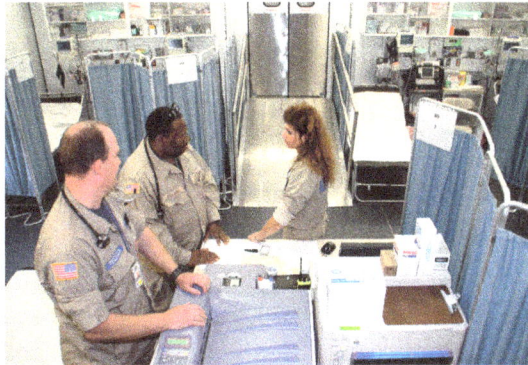

The emergency room is often a frontline venue for the delivery of primary medical care

Primary Care

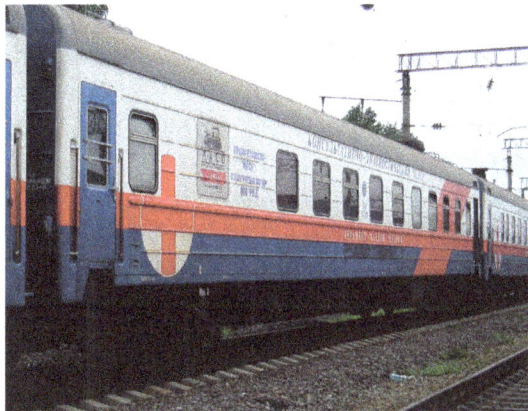

Medical train "Therapist Matvei Mudrov" in Khabarovsk, Russia

Primary care refers to the work of health professionals who act as a first point of consultation for all patients within the health care system. Such a professional would usually be a primary care physician, such as a general practitioner or family physician, a licensed independent practitioner such as a physiotherapist, or a non-physician primary care provider (mid-level provider) such as a physician assistant or nurse practitioner. Depending on the locality, health system organization, and sometimes at the patient's discretion, they may see another health care professional first, such as a pharmacist, a nurse (such as in the United Kingdom), a clinical officer (such as in parts of Africa), or an Ayurvedic or other traditional medicine professional (such as in parts of Asia). Depending on the nature of the health condition, patients may then be referred for secondary or tertiary care.

Primary care is often used as the term for the health care services which play a role in the local community. It can be provided in different settings, such as Urgent care centres which provide services to patients same day with appointment or walk-in bases.

Primary care involves the widest scope of health care, including all ages of patients, patients of all socioeconomic and geographic origins, patients seeking to maintain optimal health, and patients with all manner of acute and chronic physical, mental and social health issues, including multiple chronic diseases. Consequently, a primary care practitioner must possess a wide breadth of knowledge in many areas. Continuity is a key characteristic of primary care, as patients usually prefer to consult the same practitioner for routine check-ups and preventive care, health education, and every time they require an initial consultation about a new health problem. The International Classification of Primary Care (ICPC) is a standardized tool for understanding and analyzing information on interventions in primary care by the reason for the patient visit.

Common chronic illnesses usually treated in primary care may include, for example: hypertension, diabetes, asthma, COPD, depression and anxiety, back pain, arthritis or thyroid dysfunction. Primary care also includes many basic maternal and child health care services, such as family planning services and vaccinations. In the United States, the 2013 National Health Interview Survey found that skin disorders (42.7%), osteoarthritis and joint disorders (33.6%), back problems (23.9%), disorders of lipid metabolism (22.4%), and upper respiratory tract disease (22.1%, excluding asthma) were the most common reasons for accessing a physician.

In the United States, primary care physicians have begun to deliver primary care outside of the managed care (insurance-billing) system through direct primary care which is a subset of the more familiar concierge medicine. Physicians in this model bill patients directly for services, either on a pre-paid monthly, quarterly, or annual basis, or bill for each service in the office. Examples of direct primary care practices include Foundation Health in Colorado and Qliance in Washington.

In context of global population aging, with increasing numbers of older adults at greater risk of chronic non-communicable diseases, rapidly increasing demand for primary care services is expected in both developed and developing countries. The World Health Organization attributes the provision of essential primary care as an integral component of an inclusive primary health care strategy.

Secondary Care

Secondary care includes acute care: necessary treatment for a short period of time for a brief but serious illness, injury or other health condition, such as in a hospital emergency department. It also includes skilled attendance during childbirth, intensive care, and medical imaging services.

The term "secondary care" is sometimes used synonymously with "hospital care". However, many secondary care providers do not necessarily work in hospitals, such as psychiatrists, clinical psychologists, occupational therapists, most dental specialties or physiotherapists (physiotherapists are also primary care providers, and a referral is not required to see a physiotherapist), and some primary care services are delivered within hospitals. Depending on the organization and policies of the national health system, patients may be required to see a primary care provider for a referral before they can access secondary care.

For example, in the United States, which operates under a mixed market health care system, some physicians might voluntarily limit their practice to secondary care by requiring patients to see a primary care provider first, or this restriction may be imposed under the terms of the payment agreements in private or group health insurance plans. In other cases medical specialists may see patients without a referral, and patients may decide whether self-referral is preferred.

In the United Kingdom and Canada, patient self-referral to a medical specialist for secondary care is rare as prior referral from another physician (either a primary care physician or another specialist) is considered necessary, regardless of whether the funding is from private insurance schemes or national health insurance.

Allied health professionals, such as physical therapists, respiratory therapists, occupational therapists, speech therapists, and dietitians, also generally work in secondary care, accessed through either patient self-referral or through physician referral.

Tertiary Care

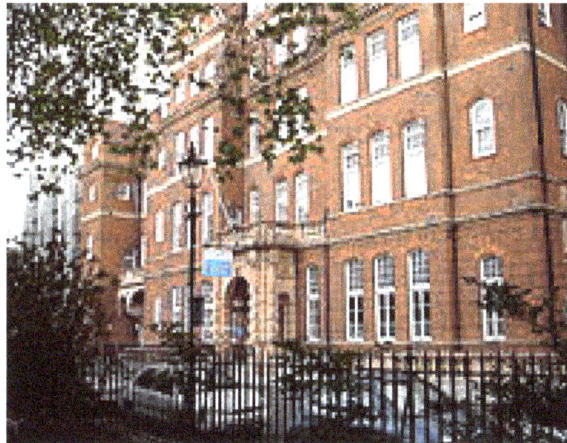

The National Hospital for Neurology and Neurosurgery in London, United Kingdom is a specialist neurological hospital.

Tertiary care is specialized consultative health care, usually for inpatients and on referral from a primary or secondary health professional, in a facility that has personnel and facilities for advanced medical investigation and treatment, such as a tertiary referral hospital.

Examples of tertiary care services are cancer management, neurosurgery, cardiac surgery, plastic surgery, treatment for severe burns, advanced neonatology services, palliative, and other complex medical and surgical interventions.

Quaternary Care

The term quaternary care is sometimes used as an extension of tertiary care in reference to advanced levels of medicine which are highly specialized and not widely accessed. Experimental medicine and some types of uncommon diagnostic or surgical procedures are considered quaternary care. These services are usually only offered in a limited number of regional or national health care centres. This term is more prevalent in the United Kingdom, but just as applicable in the United States. A quaternary care hospital may have virtually any procedure available, whereas a tertiary care facility may not offer a sub-specialist with that training.

Home and Community Care

Many types of health care interventions are delivered outside of health facilities. They include many interventions of public health interest, such as food safety surveillance, distribution of condoms and needle-exchange programmes for the prevention of transmissible diseases.

They also include the services of professionals in residential and community settings in support of self care, home care, long-term care, assisted living, treatment for substance use disorders and other types of health and social care services.

Community rehabilitation services can assist with mobility and independence after loss of limbs or loss of function. This can include prosthesis, orthotics or wheelchairs.

Many countries, especially in the west are dealing with aging populations, and one of the priorities of the health care system is to help seniors live full, independent lives in the comfort of their own homes. There is an entire section of health care geared to providing seniors with help in day-to-day activities at home, transporting them to doctor's appointments, and many other activities that are so essential for their health and well-being. Although they provide home care for older adults in cooperation, family members and care workers may harbor diverging attitudes and values towards their joint efforts. This state of affairs presents a challenge for the design of ICT for home care.

With obesity in children rapidly becoming a major concern, health services often set up programs in schools aimed at educating children in good eating habits; making physical education compulsory in school; and teaching young adolescents to have positive self-image.

Ratings

Health care ratings are ratings or evaluations of health care used to evaluate process of care, healthcare structures and/or outcomes of a healthcare services. This information is translated into report cards that are generated by quality organizations, nonprofit, consumer groups and media. This evaluation of quality can be based on:

- Measures of Hospital quality
- Measures of Health Plan Quality
- Measures of Physician Quality
- Measures of Quality for Other Health Professionals
- Measures of Patient Experience

Related Sectors

Health care extends beyond the delivery of services to patients, encompassing many related sectors, and set within a bigger picture of financing and governance structures.

Health System

A health system, also sometimes referred to as health care system or healthcare system is the organization of people, institutions, and resources to deliver health care services to meet the health needs of target populations.

Health Care Industry

The health care industry incorporates several sectors that are dedicated to providing health care services and products. As a basic framework for defining the sector, the United Nations' International Standard Industrial Classification categorizes health care as generally consisting of hospital activities, medical and dental practice activities, and "other human health activities". The last class involves activities of, or under the supervision of, nurses, midwives, physiotherapists, scientific or diagnostic laboratories, pathology clinics, residential health facilities, patient advocates, or other allied health professions, e.g. in the field of optometry, hydrotherapy, medical massage, yoga therapy, music therapy, occupational therapy, speech therapy, chiropody, homeopathy, chiropractics, acupuncture, etc.

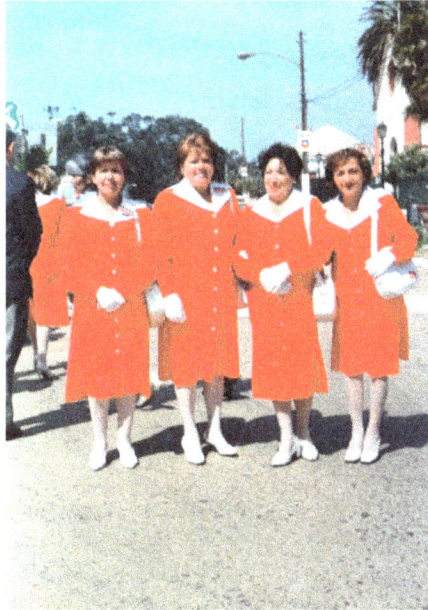

A group of Chilean 'Damas de Rojo' volunteering at their local hospital

In addition, according to industry and market classifications, such as the Global Industry Classification Standard and the Industry Classification Benchmark, health care includes many categories of medical equipment, instruments and services as well as biotechnology, diagnostic laboratories and substances, and drug manufacturing and delivery.

For example, pharmaceuticals and other medical devices are the leading high technology exports of Europe and the United States. The United States dominates the biopharmaceutical field, accounting for three-quarters of the world's biotechnology revenues.

Health Care Research

The quantity and quality of many health care interventions are improved through the results of science, such as advanced through the medical model of health which focuses on the eradication of illness through diagnosis and effective treatment. Many important advances have been made through health research, including biomedical research and pharmaceutical research, which form the basis for evidence-based medicine and evidence-based practice in health care delivery.

For example, in terms of pharmaceutical research and development spending, Europe spends a little less than the United States (€22.50bn compared to €27.05bn in 2006). The United States accounts for 80% of the world's research and development spending in biotechnology.

In addition, the results of health services research can lead to greater efficiency and equitable delivery of health care interventions, as advanced through the social model of health and disability, which emphasizes the societal changes that can be made to make population healthier. Results from health services research often form the basis of evidence-based policy in health care systems. Health services research is also aided by initiatives in the field of AI for the development of systems of health assessment that are clinically useful, timely, sensitive to change, culturally sensitive, low burden, low cost, involving for the patient and built into standard procedures.

Health Care Financing

There are generally five primary methods of funding health care systems:

1. general taxation to the state, county or municipality

2. social health insurance

3. voluntary or private health insurance

4. out-of-pocket payments

5. donations to health charities

In most countries, the financing of health care services features a mix of all five models, but the exact distribution varies across countries and over time within countries. In all countries and jurisdictions, there are many topics in the politics and evidence that can influence the decision of a government, private sector business or other group to adopt a specific health policy regarding the financing structure.

For example, social health insurance is where a nation's entire population is eligible for health care coverage, and this coverage and the services provided are regulated. In almost every jurisdiction with a government-funded health care system, a parallel private, and usually for-profit, system is allowed to operate. This is sometimes referred to as two-tier health care or universal health care.

For example, in Poland, the costs of health services borne by the National Health Fund (financed by all citizens that pay health insurance contributions) in 2012 amounted to 60.8 billion PLN (approximately 20 billion USD). The right to health services in Poland is granted to 99.9% of the population (also registered unemployed persons and their spouses).

Health Care Administration and Regulation

The management and administration of health care is another sector vital to the delivery of health care services. In particular, the practice of health professionals and operation of health care institutions is typically regulated by national or state/provincial authorities through appropriate regulatory bodies for purposes of quality assurance. Most countries have credentialing staff in regulatory boards or health departments who document the certification or licensing of health workers and their work history.

Health Information Technology

Health information technology (HIT) is "the application of information processing involving both computer hardware and software that deals with the storage, retrieval, sharing, and use of health care information, data, and knowledge for communication and decision making." Technology is a broad concept that deals with a species' usage and knowledge of tools and crafts, and how it affects a species' ability to control and adapt to its environment. However, a strict definition is elusive; "technology" can refer to material objects of use to humanity, such as machines, hardware or utensils, but can also encompass broader themes, including systems, methods of organization, and techniques. For HIT, technology represents computers and communications attributes that can be networked to build systems for moving health information. Informatics is yet another integral aspect of HIT.

Health information technology can be divided into further components like Electronic Health Record (EHR), Electronic Medical Record (EMR), Personal Health Record (PHR), Practice Management System (PMS), Health Information Exchange (HIE) and many more. There are multiple purposes for the use of HIT within the health care industry. Further, the use of HIT is expected to improve the quality of health care, reduce medical errors, improve the health care service efficiency and reduce health care costs.

Health Professional Requisites

Health professional requisites refer to the regulations used by countries to control the quality of health workers practicing in their jurisdictions and to control the size of the health labour market. They include licensure, certification and proof of minimum training for regulated health professions.

In the health care system, an health professional who offers medical, nursing or other types of health care services is required to meet specific requisites put into effect by laws governing health care practices. The number of professions subject to regulation, the requisites for an individual to receive professional licensure or certification, the scope of practice that is permitted for the individual to perform, and the nature of sanctions that can be imposed for failure to comply vary across jurisdictions.

Most countries have credentialing staff in regulatory boards or health departments who document the certification or licensing of health workers and their work history. The processes for professional certification and licensure vary across professions and countries. Certification to practise a profession usually does not need to be renewed, while a licence usually needs to be periodically renewed based on certain criteria such as passing a renewal exam, demonstrating continuing learning, being employed in the field or simply paying a fee. Most health care industry employers publish the specific requisites for persons seeking employment by means of job boards, ads and solicitations for employment. Practicing health care without the appropriate license is generally a crime.

Medical Practice Requisites

Most countries require individuals to demonstrate proof of graduation from a recognized medical school, such as one meeting the quality assurance standards of the World Federation of Medical Education, as requisite to obtain professional certification for practice as a physician or physician assistant.

In the United States, once obtaining the appropriate medical degree, physicians can apply to attain licensure via Board certification.

In India, practitioners of both modern medicine and traditional medicine are subject to professional regulation. Doctors are regulated by the Medical Council of India, while practitioners of Ayurved, Siddha and Unani medicine are regulated by the Central Council of Indian Medicine.

Nursing Requisites

Registered nurses and licensed practical nurses (or the equivalent national titles, e.g. enrolled nurses) must typically complete nursing school and pass a national examination in order to obtain their license. For example, in the United States, nurses must pass the National Council Licensure EXamination (NCLEX). They must then obtain a nursing license by applying to appropriate board of nursing. In Uganda, nurses must complete a Bachelor of Science or other diploma in nursing recognized by the Nurses and Midwives Council and pass national qualifying examinations; several years of work experience in a hospital or other health unit is further required in order to be eligible for a licence to engage in private practice.

The legal requisites as well as scope of practice for nurses (and also midwives and nurse-midwives) vary across countries. For instance, in some countries nurses are trained and authorized to provide emergency childbirth care, including administration of oxytocins and newborn resuscitation, whereas in other countries these clinical functions are only authorized for physicians.

Respiratory Therapy Requisites

Respiratory Therapists or Respiratory Care Practitioners in many countries are required to have graduated from an accredited and recognized college or university and additionally pass a registry exam prior to being eligible for licensure. In the United States, Respiratory Therapists are granted either Registry or Certificate credentials by the National Board for Respiratory Care (NBRC). The credential granted by the NBRC must be maintained to continue to hold a state licence to practice, and a fee must be paid every two years to the NBRC to maintain that credential.

Other Professional Requisites

Dentists and many other categories of allied health professions typically also require professional certification or licensure for legal practice. Training and knowledge in basic life support is required by regulation for certification for many practicing individuals, including emergency medical technicians.

Requisites and regulations for other professions, such as paramedics, clinical officers, dietitians, and homeopaths, vary across countries. They may also vary over time within countries. For example, previously no academic qualifications were needed to work as a Dental nurse in the United Kingdom; however now, hospitals, community dental services and other employers require all Dental nurses to have obtained recognized qualifications and be registered with the General Dental Council.

Practicing without a License

Practicing without a license is typically illegal. In most jurisdictions, individuals found to be providing medical, nursing or other professional services without the appropriate certification or licence may face sanctions including even criminal charges leading to prison. The number of professions subject to regulation and nature of sanctions that can be imposed for failure to comply vary across jurisdictions.

For instance, in the United States, under Michigan state laws, an individual is guilty of a felony if he practices or holds himself out as practicing a health profession subject to regulation without a license or registration or under a suspended, revoked, lapsed, void, or fraudulently obtained license or registration, or exceeding what a limited license or registration allows, or who uses the license or registration of another person as his own. The "practice of medicine" may be defined as any diagnosis, treatment, prevention, cure, or relieving of a human disease, ailment, defect, complaint, or other physical or mental condition, by attendance, advice, device, diagnostic test, or other means, or offering, undertaking, attempting to do, or holding oneself out as able to do, any of these acts.

According to the MDCH the following professions must be licensed for practice in Michigan:

• Acupuncture	• Medicine	• Podiatric Medicine & Surgery
• Athletic Trainer	• Nurse Aide	• Psychology
• Audiologist	• Nursing	• Respiratory Care
• Body Art	• Nursing Home Administrator	• Sanitarian
• Chiropractic	• Occupational Therapy	• Social Worker
• Counseling	• Optometry	• Speech-Language Pathology
• Dentistry	• Osteopathic Medicine & Surgery	• Veterinary Medicine
• Dietetics and Nutrition	• Pharmacy	
• Marriage & Family Therapy	• Physical Therapy	
• Massage Therapy	• Physician Assistant	

In Florida, such crime is classified as a third degree felony, which may give imprisonment up to five years. Practicing a health care profession without a license which results in serious bodily injury classifies as a second degree felony, providing up to 15 years' imprisonment.

In the United Kingdom, healthcare professionals are regulated by the state; the Council for Healthcare Regulatory Excellence oversees the work of various regulatory bodies including the Nursing and Midwifery Council, the General Dental Council, and the Health Professions Council (HPC). Each Council protects the 'title' of each profession it regulates. For example, it is illegal for someone to call themself an Occupational Therapist or Radiographer if they are not on the register held by the HPC.

Similarly, in South Africa, at least 12 professional titles are protected by law, subject to regulation by the Health Profession Council of South Africa.

In Uganda, a person who calls themself a "nurse" or "midwife" without having the appropriate licence from the Nurses and Midwives Council can be subject to a fine and/or up to three years of imprisonment.

Nurse Education

Nurse education consists of the theoretical and practical training provided to nurses with the purpose to prepare them for their duties as nursing care professionals. This education is provided to nursing students by experienced nurses and other medical professionals who have qualified or experienced for educational tasks. Most countries offer nurse education courses that can be relevant to general nursing or to specialized areas including mental health nursing, pediatric nursing and post-operatory nursing. Courses leading to autonomous registration as a nurse typically last four years. Nurse education also provides post-qualification courses in specialist subjects within nursing.

Historical Background

During past decades, the changes in education have replaced the more practically focused, but often ritualistic, training structure of conventional preparation. Nurse education integrates today a broader awareness of other disciplines allied to medicine, often involving inter-professional education, and the utilization of research when making clinical and managerial decisions. Orthodox training can be argued to have offered a more intense practical skills base, but emphasized the handmaiden relationship with the physician. This is now outmoded, and the impact of nurse education is to develop a confident, inquiring graduate who contributes to the care team as an equal. In some countries, not all qualification courses have graduate status.

Traditionally, from the times prior to Florence Nightingale, nursing was seen as an apprenticeship, often undertaken in religious institutes such as convents by young women, although there has always been a proportion of male nurses, especially in mental health services. In 1860 Nightingale set up the first nurse training school at St Thomas' Hospital, London. Nightingale's curriculum was largely base around nursing practice, with instruction focused upon the need for hygiene and task competence. Her methods are reflected in her *Notes on Nursing*, (1898).

Some other nurses at that time, notably Ethel Gordon Fenwick, were in favor of formalized nursing registration and curricula that were formally based in higher education and not within the confines of hospitals.

Nurse education in the United States is conducted within university schools, although it is unclear who offered the first degree level program. So far as known Yale School of Nursing became the first autonomous school of nursing in the United States in 1923.

In November 1955, a World Health Organization (WHO) study group on the education of nurses met in Brussels and made several recommendations, including that "At least one experimental school of nursing be set up in each country." In the UK, the first department of Nursing Studies at the University of Edinburgh was established in 1956, with a five-year integrated degree programme introduced in 1960. Several other universities across the UK during the 1960s. In 1974 La Trobe University commenced the very first nursing course in Australia.

Nursing Qualifications

There are multiple entry levels into nursing. This has led to confusion for the public, as well as other healthcare professionals. The earliest schools of nursing offered a Diploma in Nursing and not an actual academic degree. Community colleges began offering an Associate of Science in Nursing degree, and some diploma programs switched to this model. Universities then began to offer Bachelor of Science in Nursing and Bachelor of Nursing degrees, followed by Master of Science in Nursing degrees, and Doctor of Nursing Practice degrees.

Nursing Degrees in the UK

Pre-registration nurse training and education in the UK is now via a bachelor's degree (a UK Level 6 qualification) following the phasing-out of the Diploma of Higher Education (a UK Level 5 qualification) in Nursing which was previously offered at universities and colleges.

To become a student nurse, individuals must apply through the University and Colleges Admissions Service (commonly referred to as "UCAS") to their nursing degree choices, choosing from one of the four nursing fields: Adult, Children, Mental Health and Learning Disabilities. Requirements for entry to a pre-reg nursing degree are usually five GCSEs (including mathematics, English language and at least one science subject) at Grade C or above, along with three A-Level subjects (preferably but not essentially science-based) at Grade C or above, although the majority of universities will seek higher grades due to the competition for places. Key Skills courses are generally no-longer accepted as an alternative to GCSEs, however science or healthcare-based BTEC Level 3 Extended Diplomas and Access courses are most oftem accepted in lieu of A-Level qualifications.

If successful following interview, the student will study a "core" first year, learning basic nursing competencies essential to all four of the above fields. It is then from second year and onwards that the degree will begin to focus on the student's chosen field. Following completion of the degree, the applicant will be registered with the Nursing and Midwifery Council (NMC) as a Registered Nurse in their field of practice, using the post-nominal RNA, RNC, RNMH or RNLD as appropriate to their degree qualification.

Nursing Degrees in Western Australia

There are two specific pathways individuals can take if they wish to become a nurse in Western Australia (WA). They can decide to study at university to become a registered nurse (RN), alternatively they can study at Technical and Further Education (TAFE) to become an enrolled nurse (EN). Both pathways require a variety of entry requirements whether it be passing year 12 Maths, English and Human Biology along with receiving a specific Australian Tertiary Admission Rank (ATAR) also known as a score for university or providing prior learning experiences and legal clearances for TAFE. Either way individuals need to be aware these requirements can vary year to year and that is why they are recommended to contact each university or institute to find out entry requirements.

In WA there are four universities where individuals can choose to attend if they are wanting to complete a nursing degree.

Edith Cowan University (ECU) is located at Joondalup and South West (Bunbury) campus. ECU offers the Bachelor of Science (Nursing) degree which individuals can choose to study for three years full time or six years part time both on campus.

Curtain University is located in Bently, WA. This university offers an Undergraduate Nursing degree additionally referred to as Bachelor of Science (Nursing). This degree runs on campus for three and a half years full time however, students can request to study this degree part time.

Murdoch University also offers offer a Bachelor of Nursing degree with a three year completion date. The university offers this degree at Peel or South Street campus in Murdoch, WA.

The final university that offers a nursing degree in WA is located throughout Fremantle and is known as the University of Notre Dame. This university offer a Bachelor of Nursing degree which will take three years to achieve.

When students graduate from one of the four universities listed above they will be fully qualified as an RN and have a wide variety of job opportunities available. However, if individuals discover that university is not for them or can not gain entry into university, it is not the end of the world because there are alternative pathways available.

Attending TAFE is an alternative career pathway for individuals that still wish to pursue this profession. There are six institutes spread across WA which offer a Diploma of Nursing (Enrolled-Division 2 Nursing). These institutes include C.Y.O'Connor Institute, Great Southern Institute of Technology, Goldfields Institute of Technology, Pilbara Institute, South West Institute of Technology and West Coast Institute of Training. All institutes in WA roughly take eighteen months to complete the diploma when studying full time. Once a student successfully graduates from the Diploma of Nursing (Enrolled-Division 2 Nursing) they will be qualified as an EN.

Overall, there are alternative pathways available however an RN holds higher qualifications than an EN. There are key similarities of an RN and an EN as they both desire to fulfil their dreams of becoming a nurse and they must be registered with the Nursing and Midwifery Board of Australia, by complying with the Board's registration standards.

Scope

Nursing education includes instruction in topic areas. These are nursing assessment, nursing diagnosis, and nursing care planning. In the United States, nursing students learn through traditional classroom and lab instruction. Nursing education also involves clinical rotations and simulation, throughout their schooling, to develop care planning and clinical reasoning. At the end of schooling, nursing students in the US and Canada, must take and pass the NCLEX, National Council of Licensure Examination to practice.

Nursing Specialties

There are a variety of areas where nurses can specialise in and they may decide they want to be qualified in one or several specialities over the course of their career. Here are an array of some of the nursing specialty fields available:

- Burn Care Nurse
- Cardiology (heart) Nurse
- Clinical Nurse
- Community Health Nurse

- Mental Health Nurse
- Midwife
- Neonatal Intensive Care Nurse
- Nurse Educator

- Continence Nurse
- Diabetes Education Nurse
- District Nurse
- Dialysis Nurse
- Education
- Emergency Nurse
- Family Health Nurse
- Fertility Nurse
- Gerontology (aged care) Nurse
- Infection control
- Intensive Care
- Management
- Medical Nurse
- Nurse Manager
- Nurse Practitioner
- Occupational Health Nurse
- Oncology Nurse
- Paediatric Nurse
- Peri-operative Nurse
- Plastic Surgery Nurse
- Practice Nurse (Medical Clinic)
- Rehabilitation Nurse
- Remote Area Nurse
- Research
- Rural Nurse
- School Nurse
- Sexual Health Nurse
- Surgical Nurse
- Wound Management

Present Aims

Among nurse educators, arguments continue about the ideal balance of practical preparation and the need to educate the future practitioner to manage healthcare and to have a broader view of the practice. To meet both requirements, nurse education aims to develop a lifelong learner who can adapt effectively to changes in both the theory and practice of nursing.

While it is clear that the use of Medical simulation in nursing education is important for improving practice, patient safety, and interprofessional team skills, the balance of simulation to clinical time remains in the hands of the institutions.

Nurse Educator

A nurse educator is a nurse who teaches and prepares licensed practical nurses (LPN) and registered nurses (RN) for entry into practice positions. They can also teach in various patient care settings to provide continuing education to licensed nursing staff. Nurse Educators teach in graduate programs at Master's and doctoral level which prepare advanced practice nurses, nurse educators, nurse administrators, nurse researchers, and leaders in complex healthcare and educational organizations.

The type of degree required for a nurse educator may be dependent upon the governing nurse practice act or upon the regulatory agencies that define the practice of nursing. In the United States, one such agency is the National Council of State Boards of Nursing. For instance, faculty in the U.S. may be able to teach in an LPN program with an associate degree in nursing. Most baccalaureate and higher degree programs require a minimum of a graduate degree and prefer the doctorate for full-time teaching positions. Many nurse educators have a clinical specialty background blended with coursework in education. Many schools offer the Nurse Educator track which focuses on educating nurses going into any type setting. Individuals may complete a post-Master's certificate in education to complement their clinical expertise if they choose to enter a faculty role.

Nurse educators can choose to teach in a specialized field of their choosing. There is not extra degree needed to be earned other than a Master's degree in nursing. Most schools will only hire a nurse to teach a class if they have had experience in that area. This is so the students can have a better understanding of the current subject being taught.

In Australia, Nurse Educators must be Registered Nurses (RNs/Division 1 Nurses). The Nurse Educator role is not available to Enrolled Nurses (ENs/Division 2 Nurses). Nurse Educators require a minimum of a Certificate IV in Training and Assessment to teach the Diploma of Nursing in both the classroom and clinical placement settings. Bachelor of Nursing Educators do not technically require this qualification, but it is generally favoured. A Nurse Educator may also complete post-graduate university study in Nursing or Clinical Education, which may lead to an academic career including research, lecturing or doctoral study. To become a Clinical Nurse Educator in a healthcare setting (e.g on an acute care ward), Registered Nurses are generally required to have 5-10 years clinical experience and 6-8 years of study (a bachelor degree plus post-graduate certificate or diploma).

Critical Care Nursing

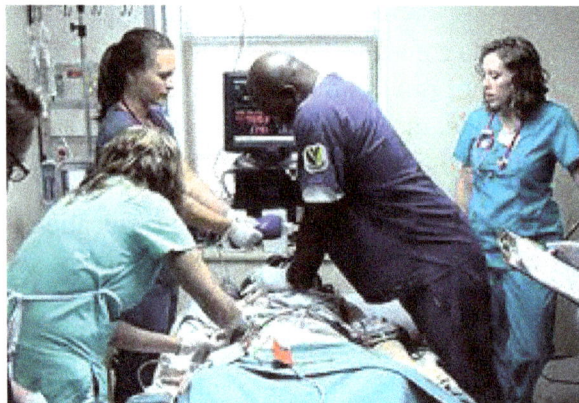

This image indicates the traumatic and stressful environment a Critical Care Nurse works in.

Critical care nursing is the field of nursing with a focus on the utmost care of the critically ill or unstable patients following extensive injury, surgery or life threatening diseases. Critical care nurses can be found working in a wide variety of environments and specialties, such as general intensive care units, medical intensive care units, surgical intensive care units, trauma intensive care units, coronary care units, cardiothoracic intensive care units, burns unit, paediatrics and some trauma center emergency departments. These specialists generally take care of critically ill patients who require mechanical ventilation by way of endotracheal intubation and/or titratable vasoactive intravenous medications.

Specific Jobs and Personal Qualities

Critical care nurses are also known as ICU nurses. They treat patients who are chronically ill or at risk for deadly illnesses. ICU nurses apply their specialized knowledge base to care for and maintain the life support of critically ill patients who are often on the verge of death. On a day-to-day basis a critical care nurse will commonly, "perform assessments of critical conditions, give intensive therapy and intervention, advocate for their patients, and operate/maintain life support systems which include mechanical ventilation via endotracheal, tracheal, or nasotracheal intubation, and titration of continuous vasoactive intravenous medications in order to maintain a " mean arterial pressure that ensures adequate organ and tissue perfusion.

Training and Education

Critical care nurses in the U.S. are trained in advanced cardiac life support (ACLS), and many earn certification in acute and critical care nursing (CCRN) through the American Association of Critical–Care Nurses. Due to the unstable nature of the patient population, LPN/LVNs are rarely utilized in a primary care role in the intensive care unit. However, with proper training and experience LPN/LVNs can play a significant role in providing exceptional bedside care for the critically ill patient. To become a critical care nurse, one must first achieve an associate or bachelor's degree in nursing and pass the National Council Licensure Examination (NCLEX-RN). Once the exam is passed, then someone can start working as a regular registered nurse (RN). After getting hired into a critical care area, additional specialized training is usually given to the nurse. After 1750 hours of providing direct bedside care in a critical care area, a nurse can then sit for the CCRN exam. The American Association of Critical Care Nurses advisory board sets and maintains standards for critical care nurses. The certification offered by this board is known as CCRN. Depending on the hospital and State, the RN will be required to take a certain amount of continuing education hours to stay up to date with the current technologies and changing techniques.

Registration is a regulatory term for the process that occurs between the individual nurse and the state in which the nurse practices. All nurses in the US are registered as nurses without a specialty. The CCRN is an example of a post registration specialty certification in critical care. There are also variants of critical care certification test that the AACN offers to allow nurses to certify in progressive care (PCCN), cardiac medicine (CMC) and cardiac surgery (CSC). In addition, Clinical Nurse Specialists can certify in adult, neonatal and pediatric acute and critical care (CCNS). In November 2007, the AACN Certification Corporation launched the ACNPC, an advanced practice certification examination for Acute Care Nurse Practitioners . None of these certifications confer any additional practice privileges, as nursing practice is regulated by the individual's state board of nursing. These certifications are not required to work in an intensive care unit, but are encouraged by employers, as the tests for these certifications tend to be difficult to pass and require an extensive knowledge of both pathophysiology and critical care medical and nursing practices. The certification, while difficult to obtain, is looked upon by many in the field as demonstrating expertise in the field of critical care nursing, and demonstrating the individual's nurse's desire to advance their knowledge base and skill set, thereby allowing them to better care for their patients.

Intensive care nurses are also required to be comfortable with a wide variety of technology and its uses in the critical care setting. This technology includes such equipment as hemodynamic and cardiac monitoring systems, mechanical ventilator therapy, intra-aortic balloon pumps (IABP), ventricular assist devices (LVAD and RVAD), continuous renal replacement equipment (CRRT/ CVVHDF), extracorporeal membrane oxygenation circuits (ECMO) and many other advanced life support devices. The training for the use of this equipment is provided through a network of in-hospital inservices, manufacturer training, and many hours of education time with experienced operators. Annual continuing education is required by most states in the U.S. and by many employers to ensure that all skills are kept up to date. Many intensive care unit management teams will send their nurses to conferences to ensure that the staff is kept up to the current state of this rapidly changing technology.

In Australia there is no compulsory prerequisite for critical care nurses to have postgraduate qualifications. However, the Australian minimum standard recommends that critical care nurses should obtain postgraduate qualifications. Critical care nurses must have a bachelor of nursing, be registered with the Nursing and Midwifery Board of Australia, and meet the NMBA's standards in order to work as a critical care nurse in Australia.

Employment Areas

Critical care nurses work in a variety of different areas, with a diverse patient population. There are many critical care nurses working in hospitals in intensive care units, post-operative care and high dependency units. They also work on medical evacuation and transport teams.

In August 2004, to demonstrate the work of critical care nurses Massachusetts General Hospital invited reporter Scott Allen and photographer Michelle McDonald from The Boston Globe to take part in an 'immersion experience' in the surgical intensive care unit (SICU). *The Globe* staffers spent eight months shadowing an experienced nurse and a trainee nurse to learn about nursing practice first hand. The result was a four-part, front-page series that ran from October 23 to 26, 2005, entitled *Critical Care: The making of an ICU nurse.*

The added psychological stress of nursing in critical care units has been well-documented, and it has been argued the stress experienced in ICU areas are unique in the profession.

Patient Interaction

According to Washington, no matter their specialty, all nurses must be able to build trusting relationships with their patients. When the nurses develop strong relationships between their patients they are able to obtain important information about them that may be helpful to diagnosing them. Also, family members that become involved in this relationship make it easier for the nurses to build these trusting relationships with the patients because the family members could ease any stress that could lead the patient to be timid. When a patient has a long-term illness, the good relationships built between the nurse and patient can improve the patient's quality of life.

Subspecialities

Critical care nurses can specialize in several different areas based on either the patient's age or the illness/injury that the patient has. Geriatric patients are considered to be people over the age of 65 and nurses that specialize in geriatrics work in an adult intensive care unit (ICU). Pediatric patients are children under the age of 18, a nurse that works with very sick children would work in a pediatric intensive care unit (PICU). Finally, a child is considered a neonatal patient from the time they are born to when they leave the hospital. If a child is born with a life-threatening illness the child would be transferred to a neonatal intensive care unit (NICU).

Also, the location that the CCRN works can vary. Some places that they can work most commonly include hospitals: in regular or specialized intensive care units. Uncommonly they can work at some patients' homes, in some flight centers and outpatient facilities.

The specialty areas of the critical care nurses can also be based on the patient's illness or injury. For example, a unit that is an adult intensive care unit, specialized in the care of trauma patients would be an adult trauma intensive care unit. The focus of the unit is generally on either an adult or a pediatric/neonatal population, as the treatment methods differ for the age ranges. Another example could include an intensive care unit solely to care for patients directly before and after a major or minor surgery.

Statistics

Depending on the location, critical care nurses work approximately 31.7 hours a week. In South Australia critical are nurses are recorded to work approximately 28.2 hours a week. While in the Northern Territory critical care nurses have been documented to work 31.7 hours a week.

Tasmania has the largest percentage of nurses working part time with 71.8%, while the Northern Territory has the lowest with 18.4%.

Salary

Critical care nurses are specialty nurses; because of this, they require more in depth and specialized training than regular RNs do. Therefore, their salaries are usually higher compared to basic RN's because of the more intense work that they do day to day. The national average salary for a CCRN is around $69,110. However, in the top percentile salaries can reach $96,630. It all depends on the job and where they are working

Critical care nurses in Australia do not need to have extra training than regular RNs do unless they have completed a postgraduate qualification. Therefore, their salaries are usually similar. Pay levels in nursing are bases on the position/level and experience. The average salary are approximately $55,617 for level 1.1, $57,841 for level 1.2, $60,155 for level 1.3, $62,561 for level 1.4, $65,063 for level 1.5, $67,666 for level 1.6, $70,373 for level 1.7, $73,187 for level 1.8, $75,488 for level 2.1, $77,028 for level 2.2, $78,600 for level 2.3 and $80,204 for level 2.4. Australian nurses receive shift loading/penalties and superannuation (approximately 10%).

Psychiatric and Mental Health Nursing

Psychiatric nursing or mental health nursing is the appointed position of a nursing that has specialized in mental health and cares for people of all ages with mental illness or mental distress, such as schizophrenia, bipolar disorder, psychosis, depression, dementia and many more. Nurses in this area receive specific training in psychological therapies, building a therapeutic alliance, dealing with challenging behavior, and the administration of psychiatric medication. A psychiatric nurse will have to have attained a bachelor's degree in nursing to become a registered nurse (RN) and specialise in mental health. Degrees vary in different countries, and are governed by country-specific regulations. Psychiatric nurses work in hospitals, mental institutes, correctional institutes, and many other facilities.

History

The history of psychiatry and psychiatric nursing, although disjointed, can be traced back to ancient philosophical thinkers. Marcus Tullius Cicero, in particular, was the first known person to create a questionnaire for the mentally ill using biographical information to determine the best course of psychological treatment and care. Some of the first known psychiatric care centers were constructed in the Middle East during the 8th century. The medieval Muslim physicians and their attendants relied on clinical observations for diagnosis and treatment.

In 13th century medieval Europe, psychiatric hospitals were built to house the mentally ill, but there were not any nurses to care for them and treatment was rarely provided. These facilities functioned more as a housing unit for the insane. Throughout the high point of Christianity in Europe, hospitals for the mentally ill believed in using religious intervention. The insane were partnered with "soul friends" to help them reconnect with society. Their primary concern was befriending the melancholy and disturbed, forming intimate spiritual relationships. Today, these soul friends are seen as the first modern psychiatric nurses.

In the colonial era of the United States, some settlers adapted community health nursing practices. Individuals with mental defects that were deemed as dangerous were incarcerated or kept in cages, maintained and paid fully by community attendants. Wealthier colonists kept their insane relatives either in their attics or cellars and hired attendants, or nurses, to care for them. In other communities, the mentally ill were sold at auctions as slave labor. Others were forced to leave town. As the population in the colonies expanded, informal care for the community failed and small institutions were established. In 1752 the first "lunatics ward" was opened at the Pennsylvania Hospital which attempted to treat the mentally ill. Attendants used the most modern treatments of the time: purging, bleeding, blistering, and shock techniques. Overall, the attendants caring for the patients believed in treating the institutionalized with respect. They believed if the patients were treated as reasonable people, then they would act as such; if they gave them confidence, then patients would rarely abuse it.

The 1790s saw the beginnings of moral treatment being introduced for people with mental distress. The concept of a safe asylum, proposed by Philippe Pinel and William Tuke, offered protection and care at institutions for patients who had been previously abused or enslaved. In the United States, Dorothea Dix was instrumental in opening 32 state asylums to provide quality care for the ill. Dix also was in charge of the Union Army Nurses during the American Civil War, caring for both Union and Confederate soldiers. Although it was a promising movement, attendants and nurses were often accused of abusing or neglecting the residents and isolating them from their families.

The formal recognition of psychiatry as a modern and legitimate profession occurred in 1808. In Europe, one of the major advocates for mental health nursing to help psychiatrists was Dr. William Ellis. He proposed giving the "keepers of the insane" better pay and training so more respectable, intelligent people would be attracted to the profession. In his 1836 publication of *Treatise on Insanity*, he openly stated that an established nursing practice calmed depressed patients and gave hope to the hopeless. However, psychiatric nursing was not formalized in the United States until 1882 when Linda Richards opened Boston City College. This was the first school specifically designed to train nurses in psychiatric care.

The discrepancy between the founding of psychiatry and the recognition of trained nurses in the field is largely attributed to the attitudes in the 19th century which opposed training women to work in the medical field.

In 1913 Johns Hopkins University was the first college of nursing in the United States to offer psychiatric nursing as part of its general curriculum. The first psychiatric nursing textbook, *Nursing Mental Diseases* by Harriet Bailey, was not published until 1920. It was not until 1950 when the National League for Nursing required all nursing schools to include a clinical experience in psychiatry to receive national accreditation. The first psychiatric nurses faced difficult working conditions. Overcrowding, under-staffing and poor resources required the continuance of custodial care. They were pressured by an increasing patient population that rose dramatically by the end of the 19th century. As a result, labor organizations formed to fight for better pay and fewer hours. Additionally, large asylums were founded to hold the large number of mentally ill, including the famous Kings Park Psychiatric Center in Long Island, New York. At its peak in the 1950s, the center housed more than 33,000 patients and required its own power plant. Nurses were often called "attendants" to imply a more humanitarian approach to care. During this time, attendants primarily kept the facilities clean and maintained order among the patients. They also carried out orders from the physicians.

In 1963, President John F. Kennedy accelerated the trend towards deinstitutionalization with the Community Mental Health Act. Also, since psychiatric drugs were becoming more available allowing patients to live on their own and the asylums were too expensive, institutions began shutting down. Nursing care thus became more intimate and holistic. Expanded roles were also developed in the 1960s allowing nurses to provide outpatient services such as counseling, psychotherapy, consultations, prescribing medications, along with the diagnosis and treatment of mental illnesses.

The first developed standard of care was created by the psychiatric division of the American Nurses Association (ANA) in 1973. This standard outlined the responsibilities and expected quality of care of nurses.

In 1975, the government published a document called "Better Services for the Mentally Ill" which reviewed the current standards of psychiatric nursing worldwide and laid out better plans for the future of mental health nursing.

Global health care underwent huge expansions in the 1980s, this was due to the governments reaction from the fast increasing demand on health care services. The expansion was continued until the economic crisis of the 1970s.

In 1982, the Area Health Authorities was terminated.

In 1983, better structure of hospitals was implemented. General managers were introduced to make decisions, thus creating a better system of operation. 1983 also saw a lot of staff cuts which was heavily felt by all the mental health nurses. However a new training syllabus was introduced in 1982, which offered suitable knowledgeable nurses.

The 2000s have seen major educational upgrades for nurses to specialise in mental health as well as various financial opportunities.

Assessment

The term mental health encompasses a great deal about a single person, including how we feel, how we behave, and how well we function. This single aspect of our person cannot be measured or easily reported but it is possible to obtain a global picture by collecting subjective and objective information to delve into a person's true mental health and well being. When identifying mental health wellness and planning interventions, here are a few things gathered from the Mental Health Association of Southern Pennsylvania to keep in mind when completing a thorough mental health assessment in the nursing profession:

- Is the patient sleeping adequate hours on a regular sleeping cycle?

- Does the patient have a lack of interest in communication with other people?

- Is the patient eating and maintaining an adequate nutritional status?

- Is the ability to perform activities of daily living present (bathing, dressing, toileting one self)?

- Can the patient contribute to society and maintain employment?

- Is the ability to reason present?

- Is safety a recurring issue?

- Does the patient often make decisions without regards to their own safety or the safety of others?

- Does the patient show a difficulty with memory or recognizance?

Interventions

Nursing interventions may be divided into the following categories:

Physical and Biological Interventions

Psychiatric Medication

Psychiatric medication is a commonly used intervention and many psychiatric mental health nurses are involved in the administration of medicines, both in oral (e.g. tablet or liquid) form or by intramuscular injection. Nurse practitioners can prescribe medication. Nurses will monitor for side effects and response to these medical treatments by using assessments. Nurses will also offer information on medication so that, where possible, the person in care can make an informed choice, using the best evidence, available.

Electroconvulsive Therapy

Psychiatric mental health nurses are also involved in the administration of the treatment of electroconvulsive therapy and assist with the preparation and recovery from the treatment, which involves an anesthesia. This treatment is only used in a tiny proportion of cases and only after all other possible treatments have been exhausted.

A patients consent to receive the treatment must be established and defended by the nurse.

Approximately 85% of clients receiving ECT have severe depression, whether seen in major depression or bipolar disorder, as the indication for use, with the remainder having another mental illness such as schizoaffective disorder, bipolar mania or schizophrenia.

Physical Care

Along with other nurses, psychiatric mental health nurses will intervene in areas of physical need to ensure that people have good levels of personal hygiene, nutrition, sleep, etc., as well as tending to any concomitant physical ailments.

Psychosocial Interventions

Psychosocial interventions are increasingly delivered by nurses in mental health settings and include psychotherapy interventions such as cognitive behavioural therapy, family therapy and less commonly other interventions such as milieu therapy or psychodynamic approaches. These interventions can be applied to a broad range of problems including psychosis, depression, and anxiety. Nurses will work with people over a period of time and use psychological methods to teach the person psychological techniques that they can then use to aid recovery and help manage any future crisis in their mental health. In practice, these interventions will be used often, in conjunction with psychiatric medications. Psychosocial interventions are based on evidence based practice and therefore the techniques tend to follow set guidelines based upon what has been demonstrated to be effective by nursing research. There has been some criticism that evidence based practice is focused primarily on quantitative research and should reflect also a more qualitative research approach that seeks to understand the meaning of people's experience.

Spiritual Interventions

The basis of this approach is to look at mental illness or distress from the perspective of a spiritual crisis. Spiritual interventions focus on developing a sense of meaning, purpose and hope for the person in their current life experience. Spiritual interventions involve listening to the person's story and facilitating the person to connect to God, a greater power or greater whole, perhaps by using meditation or prayer. This may be a religious or non-religious experience depending on the individual's own spirituality. Spiritual interventions, along with psychosocial interventions, emphasize the importance of engagement, however, spiritual interventions focus more on caring and 'being with' the person during their time of crisis, rather than intervening and trying and 'fix' the problem. Spiritual interventions tend to be based on qualitative research and share some similarities with the humanistic approach to psychotherapy.

Therapeutic Relationship

As with other areas of nursing practice, psychiatric mental health nursing works within nursing models, utilizing nursing care plans, and seeks to care for the whole person. However, the emphasis of mental health nursing is on the development of a therapeutic relationship or alliance. In practice, this means that the nurse should seek to engage with the person in care in a positive and collaborative way that will empower the patient to draw on his or her inner resources in addition to any other treatment they may be receiving.

Therapeutic Relationship Aspects of Psychiatric Nursing

The most important duty of a psychiatric nurse is to maintain a positive therapeutic relationship with patients in a clinical setting. The fundamental elements of mental health care revolve around the interpersonal relations and interactions established between professionals and clients. Caring for people with mental illnesses demands an intensified presence and a strong desire to be supportive. Dziopa and Ahern assert that there are nine critical mental health aspects of the psychiatric nursing practicum: understanding and empathy, individuality, providing support, being there/being available, being 'genuine', promoting equality, demonstrating respect, demonstrating clear boundaries, and demonstrating self-awareness for the patient.

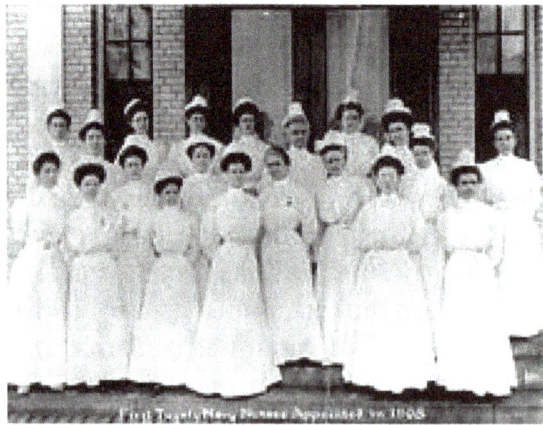

In 1913, Johns Hopkins University was the first college of nursing in the United States to offer psychiatric nursing as part of its general curriculum.

Understanding and Empathy

Understanding and empathy from psychiatric nurses reinforces a positive psychological balance for patients. Conveying an understanding is important because it provides patients with a sense of importance. The expression of thoughts and feelings should be encouraged without blaming, judging or belittling. Feeling important is significant to the lives of people who live in a structured society, who often stigmatize the mentally ill because of their disorder. Empowering patients with feelings of importance will bring them closer to the normality they had before the onset of their disorder. When subjected to fierce personal attacks, the psychiatric nurse retained the desire and ability to understand the patient. The ability to quickly empathize with unfortunate situations proves essential. Involvedness is also required when patients expect nursing staff to understand even when they are unable to express their needs verbally. When a psychiatric nurse gains understanding of the patient, the chances of improving overall treatment greatly increases.

Individuality

Individualized care becomes important when nurses need to get to know the patient. To lives this knowledge the psychiatric nurse must see patients as individual people with lives beyond their mental illness. Seeing people as individuals with lives beyond their mental illness is imperative in making patients feel valued and respected In order to accept the patient as an individual, the psychiatric nurse must not be controlled by his or her own values, or by ideas and pre-understanding of mental health patients. Individual needs of patients are met by bending the rules of standard interventions and assessment. Psychiatric/mental health nurses spoke of the potential to 'bend the rules', which required an interpretation of the unit rules and the ability to evaluate the risks associated with bending them.

Providing Support

Successful therapeutic relationships between nurses and patients need to have positive support. Different methods of providing patients with support include many active responses. Minor activities such as shopping, reading the newspaper together, or taking lunch/dinner breaks with patients can improve the quality of support provided. Physical support may also be used and is manifested through the use of touch. Patients described feelings of connection when the psychiatric nurses hugged them or put a hand on their shoulder. Psychiatric/mental health nurses in Berg and Hallberg's study described an element of a working relationship as comforting through holding a patient's hand. Patients with depression described relief when the psychiatric nurse embraced them. Physical touch is intended to comfort and console patients who are willing to embrace these sensations and share mutual feelings with the psychiatric nurses.

Being there and Being Available

In order to make patients feel more comfortable, the patient care providers make themselves more approachable, therefore more readily open to multiple levels of personal connections. Such personal connections have the ability to uplift patients' spirits and secure confidentiality. Utilization of the quality of time spent with the patient proves to be beneficial. By being available for a proper amount of time, patients open up and disclose personal stories, which enable psychiatric/mental health nurses to understand the meaning behind each story. The outcome results in nurses making every effort to attaining a non-biased point of view. A combination of being there and being available allows empirical connections to quell any negative feelings within patients.

Being Genuine

The act of being genuine must come from within and be expressed by nurses without reluctancy. Genuineness requires the psychiatric/mental health nurse to be natural or authentic in their interactions with the patient. In his article about pivotal moments in therapeutic relationships, Welch found that psychiatric nurses must be in accordance with their values and beliefs. Along with the previous concept, O'brien concluded that being consistent and reliable in both punctuality and character makes for genuinity. Schafer and Peternelj-Taylor believe that a psychiatric/mental health nurse's 'genuineness' is determined through the level of consistency displayed between their verbal and non-verbal behavior. Similarly, Scanlon found that genuineness was expressed by fulfilling intended tasks. Self disclosure proves to be the key to being open and honest. Self-disclosure involves the psychiatric/mental health nurse sharing life experiences. Self-disclosure is also essential to therapeutic relationship development because as the relationship grows patients are reluctant to give any more information if they feel the relationship is too one sided.

Multiple authors found genuine emotion, such as tearfulness, blunt feedback, and straight talk facilitated the therapeutic relationship in the pursuit of being open and honest The friendship of a therapeutic relationship is different from a sociable friendship because the therapeutic relationship friendship is asymmetrical in nature. The basic concept of genuineness is centered on being true to one's word. Patients would not trust nurses who fail in complying with what they say or promise.

Promoting Equality

For a successful therapeutic relationship to form, a beneficial co-dependency between the nurse and patient must be established. A derogatory view of the patient's role in the clinical setting dilapidates a therapeutic alliance. While patients need psychiatric/mental health nurses to support their recovery, psychiatric/mental health nurses need patients to develop skills and experience. Psychiatric nurses convey themselves as team members or facilitators of the relationship, rather than the leaders. By empowering the patient with a sense of control and involvement, psychiatric nurses encourage the patient's independence. Sole control of certain situations should not be embedded in the nurse. Equal interactions are established when psychiatric nurses talk to patients one-on-one. Participating in activities that do not make one person more dominant over the other, such as talking about a mutual interest or getting lunch together strengthen the levels of equality shared between professionals and patients. This can also create the "illusion of choice"; giving the patient options, even if limited or confined within structure.

Demonstrating Respect

To develop a quality therapeutic relationship psychiatric/mental health nurses need to make patients feel respected and important. Accepting patient faults and problems is vital to convey respect; helping the patient see themselves as worthy and worthwhile.

Demonstrating Clear Boundaries

Boundaries are essential for protecting both the patient and the psychiatric/mental health nurse and maintaining a functional therapeutic relationship. Limit setting helps to shield the patient from embarrassing behavior and instills the patient with feelings of safety and containment. Limit setting also protects the psychiatric/mental health nurse from "burnout" preserving personal stability; thus promoting a quality relationship.

Demonstrating Self-awareness

Psychiatric nurses recognize personal vulnerability in order to develop professionally. Required knowledge on humanistic, basic human values and self-knowledge improves the depth of understanding the self. Different personalities affect the way psychiatric nurses respond to their patients. The more self-aware, the more knowledge on how to approach interactions with patients. Interpersonal are skills needed to form relationships with patients were acquired through learning about oneself. Clinical supervision was found to provide the opportunity for nurses to reflect on patient relationships, to improve clinical skills and to help repair difficult relationships The reflections articulated by psychiatric nurses through clinical supervision help foster self-awareness.

Organization of Mental Health Care

Psychiatric mental health nurses work in a variety of hospital and community settings.

People generally require an admission to hospital, voluntarily or involuntarily if they are experiencing a crisis- that means they are dangerous to themselves or others in some immediate way. However, people may gain admission for a concentrated period of therapy or for respite. Despite changes in mental health policy in many countries that have closed psychiatric hospitals, many nurses continue work in hospitals though patient length of stay has decreased significantly.

Community Nurses who specialize in mental health work with people in their own homes (case management) and will often emphasize work on mental health promotion. Psychiatric mental health nurses also work in rehabilitation settings where people are recovering from a crisis episode and where the aim is social inclusion and a return to living independently in society. These nurses are sometimes referred to as *community psychiatric nurses* (the term *psychiatric* has been retained, but is being gradually replaced with the title "Community Mental Health Nurse" or CMHN)).

Psychiatric mental health nurses also work in forensic psychiatry with people who have mental health problems and have committed crimes. Forensic mental health nurses work in adult prisons, young offenders' institutions, medium secure hospitals and high secure hospitals. In addition forensic mental health nurses work with people in the community who have been released from prison or hospital and require on-going mental health service support.

People in the older age groups who are more prone to dementia tend to be cared for apart from younger adults. *Admiral Nurses* are specialist dementia nurses, working in the community, with families, carers and supporters of people with dementia. The Admiral Nurse model was established as a direct result of the experiences of family carers. The Admiral nurse role is to work with family carers as their prime focus, provide practical advice, emotional support, information and skills, deliver education and training in dementia care, provide consultancy to professionals working with people with dementia and promote best practice in person- centred dementia care.

Psychiatric mental health nurses may also specialize in areas such as drug and alcohol rehabilitation, or child and adolescent mental health.

Condition

Canada

The *registered psychiatric nurse* is a distinct nursing profession in all of the four western provinces. Such nurses carry the designation "RPN". In Eastern Canada, an Americanized system of psychiatric nursing is followed. Registered Psychiatric Nurses can also work in all three of the territories in Canada; although, the registration process to work in the territories varies as the psychiatric nurses must be licensed by one of the four provinces.

Ireland

In Ireland, mental health nurses undergo a 4-year honors degree training programme. Nurses that trained under the diploma course in Ireland can do a post graduation course to bring their status from diploma to degree.

New Zealand

Mental Health Nurses in New Zealand require a diploma or degree in nursing. All nurses are now trained in both general and mental health, as part of their three-year degree training programme. Mental health nurses are often requested to complete a graduate diploma or a post graduate certificate in mental health, if they are employed by a District Health Board. This gives additional training that is specific to working with people with mental health issues.

UK

In the UK and Ireland the term *psychiatric nurse* has now largely been replaced with *mental health nurse*. Mental health nurses undergo a 3-4 year training programme at degree level, in common with other nurses. However, most of their training is specific to caring for clients with mental health issues.

ANP (advanced nurse practitioners) - this requires completion of a masters programme. The role includes prescribing medications, assessing clients, being on call for hospital wards and delivering psychosocial interventions to clients

US

In North America, there are three levels of psychiatric nursing.

- The *licensed vocational nurse* (*licensed practical nurse* in some states) and the *licensed psychiatric technician* may dispense medication and assist with data collection regarding psychiatric and mental health clients.

- The *registered nurse* or *registered psychiatric nurse* has the additional scope of performing assessments and may provide other therapies such as counseling and milieu therapy.

- The *advanced practice registered nurse* (APRN) either practices as a clinical nurse specialist or a nurse practitioner after obtaining a master's degree in psychiatric-mental health nursing. Psychiatric-mental health nursing (PMHN) is a nursing specialty. The course work in a master's degree program includes specialty practice. APRN's assess, diagnose, and treat individuals or families with psychiatric problems/disorders or the potential for such disorders, as well as performing the functions associated with the basic level. They provide a full range of primary mental health care services to individuals, families, groups and communities, function as psychotherapists, educators, consultants, advanced case managers, and administrators. In many states, APRN's have the authority to prescribe medications. Qualified to practice independently, psychiatric-mental health APRN's offer direct care services in a variety of settings: mental health centers, community mental health programs, homes, offices, HMOs, etc.

Psychiatric nurses who earn doctoral degrees (PhD, DNSc, EdD) often are found in practice settings, teaching, doing research, or as administrators in hospitals, agencies or schools of nursing.

Australia

In Australia, to be a psychiatric nurse a bachelor's degree of nursing need to be obtained in order to become a registered nurse (RN) and this degree takes 3 years full-time. Then a diploma in mental health or something similar will need to also be obtained, this is an additional year of study. An Australian psychiatric nurse has duties that may include assessing patients who are mentally ill, observation, helping patients take part in activities, giving medication, observing if the medication is working, assisting in behaviour change programs or visiting patients who are at home. Australian nurses can work in public or private hospitals, institutes, correctional institutes, mental care facilities and homes of the patients.

References

- Adamiak, E. Chojnacka, D. Walczak, Social security in Poland – cultural, historical and economical issues, Copernican Journal of Finance & Accounting, Vol 2, No 2, p. 23

- Nadkarni, Prakash (2016). "Clinical Data Repositories: Warehouses, Registries, and the Use of Standards". Clinical Research Computing: A Practitioner's Handbook. Academic Press. pp. 173–85. ISBN 978-0-12-803145-2. doi:10.1016/B978-0-12-803130-8.00009-9

- Greengard, Samuel (1 February 2013). "A New Model for Healthcare" (PDF). Communications of the ACM. 56 (2): 1719. doi:10.1145/2408776.2408783. Retrieved 12 February 2013

- Gupta N et al. Human resources for maternal, newborn and child health: from measurement and planning to performance for improved health outcomes. Human Resources for Health 2011, 9:16 doi:10.1186/1478-4491-9-16

- O'donoghue, John; Herbert, John (2012). "Data management within mHealth environments: Patient sensors, mobile devices, and databases". Journal of Data and Information Quality (JDIQ). 4 (1): 5

- Robson, B.; Baek, O. K. (2009). The engines of Hippocrates: From the Dawn of Medicine to Medical and Pharmaceutical Informatics. Hoboken, NJ: John Wiley & Sons. ISBN 978-0-470-28953-2

- "NYU Graduate Training Program in Biomedical Informatics (BMI): A Brief History of Biomedical Informatics as a Discipline". www.nyuinformatics.org. NYU Langone Medical Center. Retrieved 11 November 2010

- Sarkar, IN (2010). "Biomedical informatics and translational medicine". J Transl Med 2010. 8: 22. doi:10.1186/1479-5876-8-22

- O'Donoghue, John; et al. (2011). "Modified early warning scorecard: the role of data/information quality within the decision making process". Electronic Journal Information Systems Evaluation. 14 (1)

- November, Joseph (2012). Biomedical Computing: Digitizing Life in the United States. Baltimore: Johns Hopkins University Press. ISBN 1421404680

- Certification Commission for Healthcare Information Technology (July 18, 2006): CCHIT Announces First Certified Electronic Health Record Products. Retrieved July 26, 2006

- Embi, PJ; Payne PR (2009). "Clinical research informatics: challenges, opportunities and definition for an emerging domain". J Am Med Inform Assoc 2009. 16 (3): 316–27. doi:10.1197/jamia.m3005

- Lussier, YA; Butte, AJ; Hunter, L (2010). "Current methodologies for translational bioinformatics.". Journal of biomedical informatics. 43 (3): 355–7. PMC 2894568. PMID 20470899. doi:10.1016/j.jbi.2010.05.002

- Collen, Morris F. A History of Medical Informatics in the United States, 1950 to 1990. Bethesda, MD: American Medical Informatics Association. ISBN 0964774305

- Slemenda, Robin (2010). "Mental Health Association of Southern Pennsylvania" (PDF). Mental Health Registered Nursing. Benedictine Home Health. Retrieved 10 May 2016

- Pyle, Kathryn I.; Lobel, Robert W.; Beck, J. Robert (1988). "Citation Analysis of the Field of Medical Decision Making". Medical Decision Making. 8 (3): 155–164. PMID 3294550. doi:10.1177/0272989X8800800302

- KQ Rao; CY Wang; JP Hu (2005). "Introduction of the National Public Health Emergency Response Information Systems Project". Chinese Journal of Integrative Medicine. 1: 2–5

- Boyd, Mary Ann; Nihart, M (1998). Psychiatric Nursing: Contemporary Practice. Philadelphia: Lippincott Williams & Wilkins. ISBN 978-0-397-55178-1

- "Clinical Informatics Board Certification" (PDF). American Board of Preventive Medicine. 1 January 2013. Retrieved 7 January 2014

- Zahabi, M. Kaber, D.B. & Swangnetr, M. (2015). Usability and safety in electronic medical records interface design: A review of recent literature. Human Factors, 57, 805-834. doi:10.1177/0018720815576827

- "Clinical Informatics 2014 Diplomats". American Board of Preventive Medicine. December 2013. Retrieved 7 January 2014

Permissions

Index